Chakras For Beginners

A Complete Guide to Balance Your Chakras and Healing Yourself with Yoga, Meditation, Crystals, Essential Oils, and Other Self-Healing Techniques

Mind, Body, and Spirit Masterclass

© Copyright 2022 - Mind, Body, and Spirit Masterclass - All rights reserved.

The following Book is reproduced below with the goal of providing information that is as accurate and reliable as possible. Regardless, purchasing this Book can be seen as consent to the fact that both the publisher and the author of this book are in no way experts on the topics discussed within and that any recommendations or suggestions that are made herein are for entertainment purposes only. Professionals should be consulted as needed prior to undertaking any of the action endorsed herein.

This declaration is deemed fair and valid by both the American Bar Association and the Committee of Publishers Association and is legally binding throughout the United States.

Furthermore, the transmission, duplication, or reproduction of any of the following work including specific information will be considered an illegal act irrespective of if it is done electronically or in print. This extends to creating a secondary or tertiary copy of the work or a recorded copy and is only allowed with the express written consent from the Publisher. All additional right reserved.

The information in the following pages is broadly considered a truthful and accurate account of facts and as such, any inattention, use, or misuse of the information in question by the reader will render any resulting actions solely under their purview. There are no scenarios in which the publisher or the original author of this work can be in any fashion deemed liable for any hardship or damages that may befall them after undertaking information described herein.

Additionally, the information in the following pages is intended only for informational purposes and should thus be thought of as universal. As befitting its nature, it is presented without assurance regarding its prolonged validity or interim quality. Trademarks that are mentioned are done without written consent and can in no way be considered an endorsement from the trademark holder.

Table of Content

Introduction 9

How Do Chakras Work? 15

The Origin of the Study of Chakras 19

The 7 Main Chakras 21

Root Chakra (1st) 29

Sacral Chakra (2nd) 35

Solar Plexus Chakra (3rd) 39

Heart Chakra (4th) 43

Throat Chakra (5th) 47

Third Eye Chakra (6th) 51

Crown Chakra (7th) 55

How to Balance and Heal Your Chakras 59

Affirmations and Mantras 63

Meditation 73

Yoga 89

Massages 95

Chromotherapy 101

Crystal Therapy 107

Essential Oils Therapy 121

The Power of Chakras: Benefits of Healthy Chakras on Physical, Mental, Emotional, and Spiritual Levels 127

Conclusion 141

Introduction

It happens to all of us, in the course of life, to face difficult times, periods of deep frustration, and sad situations that mark us deeply. At these junctures, we yearn to find the serenity and tranquility lost. To do so, we start looking for desperate solutions or magic remedies.

We look for practical remedies, then we move on to spiritual ones, but often the discomfort we feel is so deep that we do not notice that we are taking information from the wrong sources or that we are relying on the advice of unreliable people, and this only makes the situation worse.

This feeling of difficulty and discomfort that we feel inside is given by our energy that expresses itself in all its different aspects. The emotionality that we feel, the confusing feelings, the need for peace and serenity that we feel and that we are not able to reach, they all depend on our energy in that given moment.

The study of Chakras, which is the study of our energy, is the solution to understanding this feeling of emotionality and discomfort, and also to understand how this condition, in turn, causes negative consequences to our mind and then to our body.

By undertaking the study of the chakras you will no longer need to seek help from unreliable sources or wrong people. You will be able to identify for yourself the origin of your discomfort and alleviate your suffering until you eliminate it with the simple practices related to this discipline.

To understand what the Chakras are and how they work, you will have to imagine your body as a big container full of many small spheres made of energy and connected by a constant flow of energy. All these spheres are your Chakras. Among all those spheres there are 7 that are larger and have more energy than all the others, and all this energy makes them glow more than all the others. These 7 spheres are vertically aligned with each other and are the 7 Main Chakras.

The energy flowing through these spheres emits invisible but easily perceivable vibrations. Depending on the energy flowing through these spheres, the vibrations can be positive or negative.

I said that these vibrations are invisible but easily perceived and I am sure you understand exactly what I am talking about. I'm sure it has happened to you hundreds of times to enter an environment such as a room, a party hall, or a restaurant and immediately feel anxiety or discomfort, rather than joy or happiness. The people present in that environment may have a big smile on their faces, but the energy doesn't lie, and if you have felt anxiety and discomfort, those are the vibrations that those people are spreading in the environment.

I mentioned earlier that these vibrations can be positive or negative based on the energy flowing. I'm not just referring to the quality of the energy, but also to the quantity of energy. If something blocks our energy and it cannot flow freely, we experience all the various problems discussed at the beginning of this introduction: frustration, sadness, discomfort, emotionality, ... along with all the mental and physical consequences related.

Therefore, learning about your Chakras, how to unlock their energy, and how to balance it will allow you to heal these discomforts. If you make these practices of unblocking, healing, and balancing the energy of the Chakras part of your daily life, you will enjoy very long periods of well-being and you will truly never again need to go looking for magical solutions from the wrong sources.

Immerse yourself in the study of Chakras, in the study of your own energy. It will allow you to take control of your life and direct it towards the happiness and peace that you deserve and want. You can improve relationships with people you care most for and those around you. More generally, you can improve your relationship with the world around you.

In order to keep the Chakras open and functioning, it is necessary to understand what may be causing the blocks that interrupt or reduce the flow of energy. In the in-depth analysis of each of the 7 main Chakras, we will go into detail about the specific causes of blockage of each specific Chakra, but I think it is very important to illustrate what I consider a fundamental element for understanding the problem.

The causes of energy that does not flow properly or is blocked can be many. For example, having bad habits or not taking proper care of your body can be the main cause of the malfunctioning of our energy centers. There are 2 elements in particular, however, that I believe to be the major causes of

Chakras blockage: continually trying to repress yourself to be different from what you are and negativity, negative energy expressed through negative emotions.

Trying to show to be different from what you really are so that you are closer to a socially acceptable ideal causes anxiety, depression, and mental and emotional stress. All these negative feelings lead us to the second cause of Chakras' blockage.

When I speak of negative feelings or emotions, however, I am not just referring to yours. Your energy centers pick up energy from the world around you, so they also pick up the negative vibrations of the people around you who are plagued by negative emotions. As you can see, it's not just a matter of knowing how to handle your negative emotions, but more importantly, choosing well the people you surround yourself with. Doing an excellent job on yourself and then hanging out with people who radiate negativity would negate all your good work. Not only that but by associating with these people you would end up passing through or staying in places impregnated with those negative vibrations that would further block your flow of positive energy.

In the next chapters, you will understand how to work well on your Chakras but accept the advice to choose carefully the people with whom you hang around and the places you frequent.

Don't be afraid of not knowing how to choose, as you read these lines you probably already have negative places or people in mind. You know this because when you meet them you feel a sadness that you can't explain, or you reach the house of "a friend" and feel an unfounded sense of unease. Trust your energetic sphere and clean your surroundings of toxic people and places and you will see the first benefits immediately.

How Do Chakras Work?

I mentioned in the introduction that Chakras are spheres of energy connected by a constant flow of energy. But where does this energy come from? Chakras allow the energy of the external world to enter and flow within us. I used the similarity with the spheres to introduce the Chakras because the translation of the Sanskrit term is "circle" or "wheel".

You can imagine Chakras as small luminous wheels in perpetual movement that receive energy from the external world and expand it in a constant flow within each one of us. This energy flowing within each one of us, allows our body to perform all its functions on the physical level, the mental level, the spiritual level, and the emotional level, that is, on all four "layers" of the human being.

These little wheels of energy in our body, our Chakras, are hundreds in number. It is essential for our wellness on all four levels of our being that the energy that enters our body flows abundantly and constantly through all those wheels. Not all Chakras are the same, there are major and minor ones, but they must all allow the energy to flow appropriately. At the moment in which even only one of them does not carry out its function correctly, we immediately begin to experience symptoms.

Within the major and minor Chakras, we can identify seven Chakras that are called "The 7 Main Chakras". As I mentioned in the introduction, they are vertically aligned and we can visualize them in a vertical line that follows the spine from the base to the top of the head. Each of these 7 Chakras is positioned at an exact point of the spine.

You will have understood by now that our whole daily life is influenced by our Chakras and their state of health. If our energy is not flowing as it should then our life will surely have problems.

In the following chapters, we are going to analyze in deeper detail the characteristics of each one of the 7 main Chakras, their causes of blockage, how to remove those blocks, and all the information you will need to bring harmony back into your life. The first step of this process, however, is awareness and you have already walked this first step by starting to study this manual. Being aware of the existence of the Chakras and knowing how to use them to your advantage, by keeping them open so that energy can flow freely, is the first step to maintaining good physical, mental, emotional, and spiritual health.

Chakras influence our daily life so deeply because they don't just take care of the energy in our physical body, but they act as a bridge connecting our body to the mind, the emotions, and the spirit. By the terms mind, emotions and spirit I am referring to the parts of the human body that are invisible to the senses. Each Chakra must work in harmony and balance with the others to create the ideal condition for our well-being. This ideal condition is a harmonic connection between our visible and invisible parts.

Each of the 7 main Chakras has, in fact, a physical correspondent such as an organ or a gland, and also a specific correspondence to certain aspects of our "invisible part". According to the Indian tradition, from which the Chakras originate, each of the 7 main Chakras is also linked to different colors, sounds, frequencies, mantras, images, and deities and it is because of these characteristics that each Chakra affects a different area of our daily life.

We spoke before about hundreds of spheres, while now we have reduced to 7 main Chakras. There are 2 other groups of Chakras, besides the 7 main ones.

In the second group, we find the so-called Minor Chakras, mainly located in the center of the palm of the hands, in the fingertips, in the linga, in some areas of our feet, and in some other areas.

The third group of Chakras includes all those of very small size or, even, tiny. They are so many to be practically incalculable, you can find one at each point where two energy lines meet.

We will deal with the opening, balancing, and unlocking of the 7 main ones. Basically, when the 7 Chakras work in harmony with each other, the ones belonging to the second and third groups just follow along.

The Origin of the Study of Chakras

The study of Chakras and their structure has very ancient origins. The original study of Chakras has its roots in India and the oldest evidence of this study are the Vedas, an ancient collection of popular sacred texts in Sanskrit. As for the historical period, we are between 1500 and 500 B.C. and originally the study of these "wheels" was handed down orally.

Western culture came across these ancient studies in 1919 with the book of Arthur Avalon, an English student of these disciplines, entitled "The Power of the Serpent". This book is considered the first document studying the application of

Kundalini Yoga. In the work, the author describes the philosophical and mythological nature of Kundalini and explains the anatomy associated with it, i.e. the energy centers of the human body (Chakras), their progressive awakening, and the Yoga poses and techniques associated with this practice of awakening. The most interesting part strictly related to the topic we are discussing, however, is that the book contains the translation of two ancient Indian documents that, until then, were considered secret and one of them is entirely dedicated to the study of Chakras.

From this important starting point, the study of Chakras has gone from being a subject for a few enthusiasts to a discipline of study for a wider audience. Most people now find this term quite familiar and feel comfortable with the study of this discipline and the benefits that its knowledge can bring to the life of each individual.

The 7 Main Chakras

Let's briefly recap what has been said so far. Chakras are spheres of energy in our body that are responsible for letting the energy in and making it flow from one point to another. They are located in a part of the body that is not perceptible to the senses. This part is called the "astral body" and is where the soul lives. The "astral body" is a part of the "subtle bodies", which are the layers of the human body that the senses cannot see or perceive. The "subtle bodies" are energy fields composed of etheric organs that have an equivalent on the physical plane with physical organs such as the heart, the liver, and so on.

The 7 main Chakras, therefore, are located in the "astral body" along the line of the spine, and, starting from the bottom and going upwards, they run along the whole spinal column. Each of them has an equivalent organ on the physical plane, therefore an organ of our body. Each Chakra transmits a specific vibration, associated with a certain color.

With this premise, it is easy to understand how the blockage of a Chakra can cause problems on a physical, mental, spiritual, and emotional level.

The functioning of the Chakras is quite simple. They take energy from the Universe, store it and then act as crossroads for its distribution. They make it flow towards all the adjacent Chakras in a constant and regular flow. As long as this condition of flow is respected, you will feel well physically, mentally, spiritually, and emotionally.

The moment one of these energy centers is blocked, a regular and constant flow of energy in your body will no longer occur, and as a result, various physical, mental, spiritual, or emotional problems will start to show up in your life. The type of problem will depend on which Chakra is not properly open, and therefore where the blockage and misalignment originates.

How can you tell if your Chakras are aligned or not? You simply need to analyze yourself to see if you have symptoms. We will go into more detail later, but I can start to give you some suggestions. Do you ever wake up with an unexplainable feeling of discomfort and unease? Do you often feel sad for no reason? Do you often feel strong, exaggerated, and uncontrolled feelings towards someone? Are you unable to express your creativity? Do you feel like you can never have fun? Do you have low self-esteem and constant fear of rejection? Do you suffer from hard-to-justify and uncontrollable outbursts of anger? Do you find it difficult to communicate with others whether it is in words or in writing?

I could go on with the list but these first questions should be enough to make you think about your actual situation. If you find yourself in one or more of the circumstances I have just described in my questions, then it is very likely that one of your Chakras is creating a blockage to your energy flow, and so your energy cannot proceed as it should, in a flux regular and constant.

It is fundamentally important to understand this process because with the awareness you gain you can decide to take action to remove the blockage. In the course of the book, you will understand how to identify which Chakra is responsible for what distress, and how to fix the problem. I would like to anticipate, however, that there are many methods to unlock and free your energy and you can choose the one you feel is more adaptable to you. Numerous Yoga positions allow the energy to flow, opening the Chakras and regulating their flow. Some massages perform a similar function. Furthermore, since each Chakra is associated with a color, gemstone, essential oil, and a certain vibration, you could choose to unblock your Chakras and rebalance them with color therapy, essential oils, and the use of particular minerals and gems. Meditation on its own, or accompanied by the repetition of Mantras or positive affirmations is also very useful.

Now let's go a little deeper into understanding each individual Chakra.

Each Chakra rotates at a different speed and has a different brightness according to the age of a person and his physical condition. So, brightness and rotation speed change using the course of a person's life because of the increasing ages, and because of the changing conditions, for example in case of stress or disease.

We have already said several times that when we look at the position of Chakras we move from the bottom to the top. We can identify the first three at the base of our spine moving up towards the head. They are the three lowest or "inferior" ones and are those related to the material needs and the fundamental needs of the human being. Included in this group of needs are food and nourishment, protection, economic security and, therefore, money, but also self-esteem, the need to be accepted, physical appearance, and sex.

The top three, moving up from the throat, are the "upper" and "higher" ones. They are more related to spirituality and otherworldly needs. This group of needs includes the search for the reason why we come into the world, the desire to evolve and improve, the desire to understand ourselves and others, but also ambition and the search for truth as opposed to illusion.

To regulate the lower and upper Chakras there is the Heart Chakra, the center of the entire energy system, the Chakra of love in all its forms, which aims to maintain a balance between soul, mind, and body.

Before moving on to the analysis of each Chakra I would like to emphasize once again that each Chakra corresponds to an organ of our body from the anatomical point of view. This means that, if the Chakra connected to a certain organ is blocked, the organ could not function correctly and could not perform its functions in a totally correct way. This malfunctioning could potentially lead your body into a state of disease and that is why it is essential to make sure that your Chakras are always open, and well balanced. In this way, your vital energy can flow properly leading you to enjoy physical, mental, spiritual, and emotional health.

The energy that flows in our body is called "Prana" in Indian philosophical terminology. This name comes from Sanskrit, a language in which the term "Prana" means life, but is also used with the meaning of "spirit" or "breath". Therefore, "Prana" is the vital energy that flows within and around us. Thanks to the "Prana", we communicate with the outside world in a constant exchange of energy and vitality, we take energy from the world around us and return it. This energy, "Prana", is connected to our Chakras, it's the energy that flows through your Chakras.

Now let's find out what the 7 main Chakras are, what they influence, which organs of the body they are identified with, what vibration and color they correspond to, and a lot more. You need this information because it is through these "rules" that the Chakras manage your life. Your energy flow is managed according to these basic criteria. You will be able to use this information to make a "diagnosis" about the state of each one of your Chakras.

Root Chakra (1st)

(Sanskrit name: Mūlādhāra)

Element: Earth

Color: Red

Position: Coccyx

Planet: Mars

Characteristics of a well-balanced Chakra: It is called the Root Chakra because it is the root that connects us directly with the Earth, our mother. It keeps us constantly anchored to our material reality, makes us desire stability, and always have a contact and a connection with our roots. It is the Chakra of stability and is closely linked to the survival instinct and the basic needs of the human being. It is the Chakra of vitality and energy, regeneration of blood and tissues. It is responsible for giving a sense of security and stability, promoting destiny, and generating warmth. This Chakra also acts as a link with our past, our roots, and our ancestors. If it is well balanced we live our memories with harmony and without excessive attachment, we are not obsessed with the past, and we can live in the present, letting go of memories when necessary. The first Chakra gives us a strong instinct to survive and a balanced attachment to life, together with great respect for our body and our planet, necessary for our life and our survival.

Personal qualities related to this Chakra: Survival, being well-grounded, satisfaction, stability, instinctive trust, courage, vitality, power to achieve goals, full acceptance of life.

Which organs is it associated with? Spine, legs, feet, ankles, bones, coccyx, rectum, kidneys, bladder, prostate, male reproductive system, immune system, sense of smell, nose, skin, nails, teeth, and gums.

What physical problems is it related to? It is linked to physical problems that affect the intestine and the difficulty in the clearing, purifying, and eliminating toxins. There are frequent problems with the bones, legs, feet, and knees due to a bone structure that is not very solid. It is often associated with a stiff and not very fluid way of walking. It may cause problems with teeth, problems losing weight, problems with obesity, nervous anorexia, and even problems with the genital organs. Severe weakness for no reason is also common.

What part of the emotional sphere does it affect? Being this Chakra so deeply linked to human basic needs and instinct of survival, and self-preservation, it gives us the desire to live and experience the material world and what it has to offer. It makes us desire monetary autonomy, money through which we can meet the basic needs of feeding, clothing, and shelter. It makes us desire to put down roots in a place where we are happy, but it also makes us desire to change for a better and better life.

Symptoms of a blocked Chakra: First and foremost, you feel a sense of abasement and disconnection with your surroundings: you never feel at home anywhere. You feel chained to the surrounding environment, or to the people in your personal sphere because of low self-love and low self-esteem. A conflictual relationship with the mother figure is common. Usually, you never notice a specific reason as the cause of discomfort. Another symptom of the blockage of this Chakra is a strong sense of instability and difficulty in adapting to change. This internal and emotional discomfort manifests itself in some of the physical symptoms already described. Economic problems are also a clear symptom of the blockage of this Chakra, as well as doing a job that you do not like, and that does not give you stimulus or satisfaction.

Possible causes of blockage or imbalance: Too fearful or too greedy behaviors can be a primary cause. Pretending that everything is always fine, while inside we are oppressed by fear, can also be a cause of a blockage. Cultivating fear and continuing to blame ourselves for cultivating it are further obstacles to the flow of the Chakra's energy. Another cause of imbalance or blockage is the relationship between the person and his surrounding environment. In the definition of the surrounding environment, we can include all the people that revolve around the person himself, such as friends, family, partner, … If the person is inserted in an environment that is wrong for him, here we have the problems described in the symptoms of the blocked Chakra. In this regard, if you feel judged by the people who make up your surrounding environment, this can lead to problems. In fact, if you hide your nature in order not to run into these judgments you create a strong obstacle to the flow of your energy.

Gems of the Root Chakra: The gems and stones that help to balance this Chakra are those of yellow-reddish color. The main one is red jasper, but it is also in tune with red agate and fire agate, red calcite, hematite, garnets, black onyx, fire opal, obsidian, ruby, smoky quartz, and brown zircon.

Associated colors: Red, brown, black, and gray

Associated sense: Olfaction

Associated fragrances: Cedar, sandalwood, cypress, patchouli, vetiver, and olibanum. These are strong, intense fragrance oils that are dark in color and have a woody or resinous scent.

Associated number: 4

Associated mantra: LAM

Associated foods: Foods that regulate body temperature, hot and energetic foods, such as chili peppers, tomatoes, radicchio, red onions, eggs, beets, meat, ... (mainly red foods).

Sacral Chakra (2nd)

(Sanskrit Name: Svadhishthana)

Element: Water

Color: Orange

Position: Below the navel (pubis)

Planet: Mercury

Characteristics of the well-balanced Chakra: Sexual creativity, balance, serenity, joviality, and spontaneity. The second Chakra influences our relationships with others, our sexuality, our pleasure and physical well-being, and the way we manage our emotions. Its foundation is pleasure and recognition for us from others. The second Chakra offers us a deep connection of harmony with nature that we see expressed in creative activities such as gardening, painting, photography, or even martial arts. To be in harmony with this Chakra means to be at peace with yourself, at ease and aware of your strengths and weaknesses, and to be magnetic and luminous people. It is the Chakra of our social instinct, of wanting to live among more people, and not alone.

Personal qualities related to this Chakra: Primary feelings, sexuality, desire, sensuality, pleasure, relationships, admiration, union with nature, openness, transparency, and personal creativity.

Which organs is it associated with? Ovaries, testicles, reproductive system, small intestine, spleen, bladder, digestive and intestinal system, and sciatic nerve.

What physical problems is it related to? The imbalance of this Chakra is linked to sexual or reproductive problems, back pain in the pelvic area, and disorders in the kidneys and urination.

What part of the emotional sphere does it affect? This Chakra influences the ability to express love, but also one's ability to express desires, creativity, and have fun along the way. When balanced we are pervaded by creativity, confidence, and passion. It is the Chakra that is the home to all of our emotions. These emotions can be positive or negative based on previous experiences and also based on the social context, family, and friends around us.

Symptoms of a blocked Chakra: The main symptom is a lack of confidence mainly in oneself and continuous unfounded fears. There are frequent emotional blocks, low passion, absence of libido, and creativity in all its forms. For example, we fail to connect with our passions, or we lack the enthusiasm to do so. In some cases, we feel a spasmodic need to keep all aspects of our lives under control, and we lack love and self-esteem. We fail to connect with others, even in intimacy. Weakness, exhaustion, and feeling lacking in gifts or talents are all very clear symptoms of energy blockage in this Chakra. Fear, anger, and anxiety dominate us when this Chakra is not functioning well, often resulting in a sense of depression. We experience life as a kind of struggle where we are alone to face everyone, and can never find serenity.

Possible causes of blockage or imbalance: Emotional trauma, constant stress, and too sedentary life are the main causes of blockage. Feelings of guilt are another cause of strong blockage of this Chakra's energy. The feeling of guilt is associated with the feeling of being imprisoned because you don't want to take responsibility for your life and, therefore, getting rid of want doesn't do you any good. On a physical level, the blockage of energy can be caused by abuse of our body, for example, if we stress it with continuous negative thoughts, or if we mistreat it with the consumption of alcohol, and cigarettes.

Gems of the Sacral Chakra: The main gem of this Chakra is the Carnelian, the stone of mental and spiritual pleasure. It is however in tune with most stones in shades of orange such as amber, moonstone, fire opal, and orange calcite.

Associated color: Orange

Associated sense: Taste

Associated scents: Jasmine, orange, gardenia, ylang-ylang, pine, birch, and juniper. These are less strong essential oils than those of the first Chakra, with a strong aphrodisiac power, or the power to stimulate purification.

Associated number: 6

Associated mantra: VAM

Associated foods: The foods of this Chakra are those naturally sweet, rich in minerals, and aphrodisiacs such as oranges, mandarins, pumpkin, saffron, carrots, and mangoes, apricots, honey, coconut, oats, sesame, cinnamon ... (mainly orange food).

Note: the passing of too much energy through this Chakra can cause excessive lust, addiction in various forms, and an excessive sense of control. This makes it critical that the flow of energy is constantly kept balanced.

Solar Plexus Chakra (3rd)

(Sanskrit name: Manipura)

Element: Fire

Color: Yellow

Position: Above the navel

Planet: Jupiter

Characteristics of the well-balanced Chakra: This Chakra carries the power of wisdom and knowledge. It controls our ego. It makes us aware of our new physical and mental potential. It helps us to be who we really want to be. It promotes digestion and gives access to happiness and self-confidence. It allows us to assimilate energy. It gives us tranquility, respect, and dignity towards ourselves. Its main purpose is our self-acceptance. It is the Chakra responsible for our actions and our intentionality.

Personal qualities related to this Chakra: Personal power, strength, authority, self-control, peace, joy, inner harmony, self-acceptance, social identity.

Which organs is it associated with? Pancreas, nervous system, digestive system, liver, spleen, large intestine, stomach, transverse colon, gallbladder, metabolism, muscles, and eyes.

What physical problems is it related to? Disorders of the liver, stomach, pancreas, gallbladder, and colon. Ulcers and gastritis are frequent. Bloating. Problems with teeth and gums.

What part of the emotional sphere does it affect? It affects the emotional sphere of self-esteem, self-criticism, and our relationship with power.

Symptoms of a blocked Chakra: Strong selfishness, deep states of anxiety, sense of shame, and problems related to self-assertion on the physical, mental, and emotional levels. For example, it manifests in the form of a fear of rejection or criticism for one's physical appearance. This creates a tendency to isolate oneself and avoid contact with others. You feel inadequate, powerless, and unable to achieve your goals. Everything seems like an insurmountable obstacle. Anger is repressed rather than expressed, causing deep mental distress that spills over into the body causing illness.

Possible causes of blockage or imbalance: A poor care of our image could be the main cause of the imbalance of this Chakra. This is true on the outer level and it is expressed in the way we dress, in the way we take care of our bodies, and in the way we take care of our physical form. It is also true on the emotional and intellectual level and it is expressed by the fact that we don't have goals to achieve or that we don't celebrate our victories and successes. The tendency to suppress our abilities and talents can also be an obstacle to the flow of energy through this Chakra. Feelings of frustration and shame are major obstacles to its balanced energy flow. We never pause to analyze the causes of negative, deleterious, and destructive emotions, thus aggravating the blockage.

Gems of the Solar Plexus Chakra: The main stone is citrine quartz. This Chakra is however attuned to yellow stones such as gold, yellow zircon, pyrite, yellow opal, tiger's eye, imperial topaz, and sulfur.

Associated colors: Yellow and gold

Associated sense: Sight

Associated fragrances: Grapefruit, lemon, mint, cardamom, clove, coriander, cinnamon, and black pepper. These are either oils from plants that stimulate digestion or oils that are spicier and warmer.

Associated number: 10

Associated mantra: RAM

Associated Foods: This Chakra receives energy primarily from yellow-colored foods such as lemons, bananas, pineapples, peppers, wheat and cereal, ginger and turmeric, sunflower seeds, and cheese.

Heart Chakra (4th)

(Sanskrit name: Anahata)

Element: Air

Color: Green

Position: In the center of the chest

Planet: Venus

Characteristics of the well-balanced Chakra: This Chakra represents the place where love and tenderness are born. It is responsible for the balance of our emotions and our openness to life and relationships. The main purpose of this Chakra is the expression of love in all its forms and, when the energy flows correctly, we feel proud, full of pleasure, love, and trust, ready to forgive anyone. It balances the heart and mind, promotes healing, and gives a sense of calm and tranquility. It is the seat of the purest energy and feelings and acts as a bridge toward the spiritual world. When it is well balanced we feel happy and motivated.

Personal qualities related to this Chakra: Unconditioned love, healing, compassion, harmony, transformation, devotion, and sharing.

Which organs is it associated with? Heart, vagus nerve, skin, hands and arms, vertebrae, chest, bronchi and lungs, cardiovascular, respiratory, and immune systems.

What physical problems is it related to? Pain in the back, shoulders, arms, and wrists. Pulmonary problems, bronchial asthma, and cardiovascular diseases. Digestive problems and ulcers. Weak eyesight.

What part of the emotional sphere does it affect? This is the Chakra of love, forgiveness, understanding, and motivation. It influences the emotional sphere that revolves around these feelings and emotions.

Symptoms of a blocked Chakra: There is a strong fear of being alone. There are frequent bursts of anger or feelings of deep bitterness, even unjustified. In love, you tend to be suffocating and morbidly jealous. You feel pervaded by a deep sadness of which you cannot identify the cause and you feel pain because of this. You tend to become dependent on feelings and, in some way, on those around you, and on their judgment. One is afraid to commit, tends to cheat, be dishonest, and be alone.

Unhealthy relationships are a clear example of the blockage of this Chakra.

Possible causes of blockage or imbalance: This Chakra is damaged by some of the most common life experiences. For example, having received little love and care as a child and in the growth phase, for example, from an uncaring parent or parent too focused on himself. More extreme situations in childhood can also be a cause of the blockage, such as physical or emotional trauma. They could also be more recent causes such as having developed wrong ideas and beliefs about love or having undertaken bad behavioral habits that prevent giving and healthily receiving love. Blocking this Chakra are the emotional states related to the sensations of internal emotional pain.

Gems of the Heart Chakra: The main gems of this Chakra are Green Tourmaline and Rose Quartz. It is however in harmony with all the stones of green and pink color such as pink and green agate, jade, aventurine, malachite, emerald, and pink and green zircon.

Associated colors: Green and pink

Associated sense: Touch

Associated fragrances: Lavender, rose geranium, rose, lemon balm, and sweet orange. These are essential oils with softening, comforting, sedative, soothing, harmonious, and revitalizing powers.

Associated number: 12

Associated mantra: YAM

Associated foods: This Chakra draws energy from all green vegetables and those that have a green leafy plant. Especially important for the balance of this Chakra are green tea and herbs such as thyme, basil, and marjoram.

NOTE: Excessive energy flowing through this Chakra can lead to a loss of emotional control and, therefore, to the occurring of the wrong emotions at the wrong time. It is vital to take care of the balance and stability of its energy flow at all times.

Throat Chakra (5th)

(Sanskrit name: Vishuddha)

Element: Ether

Color: Blue

Position: Throat, at the intersection with the clavicle

Planet: Saturn

Characteristics of the well-balanced Chakra:
Communication, openness to others, and listening. From this Chakra enters and exits "Prana" (the energy we discussed earlier). It has the task of controlling communication and producing sounds. The produced sounds originate vibrations that put us in tune with the vibrations of the universe. It stimulates creativity and gives mental clarity. Its main purpose is to allow our inner voice to be heard. When it is perfectly balanced, we express ourselves adequately and the words come out with a constant pleasant flow. If the energy flows correctly, we are honest, sincere, and good listeners not only for others but also for ourselves. We listen without judging. Sincerity and honesty are both characteristics of this Chakra and they are both

directed toward others and ourselves. When this Chakra is in harmony, we really listen to others, to ourselves, to our thoughts, and to our desires. We create opportunities for ourselves, we develop our creative side, we become part of the world, of its universal rhythm, and we connect to others without being conditioned and crushed by their opinions.

Personal qualities related to this Chakra: Freedom, independence, expression of one's creativity, inspiration, truth, sincerity.

Which organs is it associated with? It mainly affects the metabolic system and the respiratory system with the throat, mouth, vocal cords, trachea, larynx, tonsils, bronchi, and lungs. It also affects the esophagus, cervical vertebrae, and the area of arms, shoulders, and neck.

What physical problems is it related to? You may experience thyroid problems, sore throats and chronic infections, discomfort and tension in the neck and shoulders, pain in the ear or in the area of the jaws and jaws, and dizziness and poor balance.

What part of the emotional sphere does it affect? It influences the sphere of giving voice to our emotions without fear and how this allows us to connect to others, to become part of the world, and of its rhythm. This Chakra also influences our creative side, helping us to channel our energies in the best possible way.

Symptoms of a blocked Chakra: We fail to communicate and tend to keep everything inside, including the emotions that we cannot express. We begin to reduce our contact with others, we fear new friendships, and become distrustful as if others are always ignoring our own interests. This often causes us to become manipulative towards others, even unconsciously. We become increasingly lazy, without self-esteem, and with a tendency to fall into immobility.

Possible causes of blockage or imbalance: The blockage or imbalance usually occurs when a person continues to lie to himself and to others. It also occurs when there is a lack of honesty in behaviors and attitudes, both to the detriment of oneself and others.

Gems of Throat Chakra: The main stone of this Chakra is Aquamarine. It is, however, in harmony and resonance with all blue and light blue stones: Sapphire, blue zircon, and turquoise.

Associated colors: Light blue and blue

Associated sense: Hearing

Associated fragrances: Eucalyptus, sage, bergamot, verbena, chamomile, and tea tree. These are essential oils with soothing, harmonizing power, and a balsamic effect.

Associated number: 16

Associated mantra: HAM

Associated foods: Since there are no blue foods in nature, it is difficult to energize this Chakra with food. Water, however, is important for its balance and with it all the drinks that can be made from it, such as juices, teas, infusions, and herbal teas. Algae, which grow in water, are very useful to energize this Chakra, and they are delicious to prepare your dishes.

NOTE: If the flow of energy through this Chakra is too intense, there is a risk of speaking too aggressively, and showing excessive superiority. You develop a tendency to talk too much, too fast, and always interrupt others. For this reason, it is fundamental to keep the flow of this Chakra balanced and constant at all times.

Third Eye Chakra (6th)

(Sanskrit Name: Ajna)

Element: Light

Color: Indigo

Position: Between the eyebrows

Planet: Jupiter

Characteristics of the well-balanced Chakra: Awareness is the main characteristic of the sixth Chakra. The purpose of this Chakra is to understand the bigger picture in every area. It is often associated with the acquisition of supernatural powers because the spiritual sight that it gives us, allows us to see things that escape ordinary people. This Chakra allows us to have a clear vision of what is around us, but also of what is within us. It makes us develop a strong intuition, almost always right, and deals with our communication with the subconscious, where our deepest motivations lie. It allows us to become aware of ourselves, who we really are, what we really need, and what our reality is. Thanks to the sixth Chakra, we can be centered in the here and now, we can see beyond appearances, and disengage ourselves from material possessions, the fear of death, and other paralyzing phobias. It protects us from outside influences, opens us up to and facilitates change. It helps us to develop freedom of thought and inspiration, often expressed through art forms. It makes us focused, determined, and have a clear idea of what is real, and what is illusory.

Personal qualities related to this Chakra: Intuition, clairvoyance, imagination, projection of the will, and mental peace.

Which organs is it associated with? Nose, forehead, temples, ears, left eye, nervous system, cerebellum, marrow, and hormonal system.

What physical problems is it related to? Problems of sight, hearing, sinusitis, and also hormonal dysfunctions are frequent and linked to imbalances in this Chakra.

What part of the emotional sphere does it influence? It is a Chakra strongly linked to mood, fears, and the distinction between dreams and reality.

Symptoms of a blocked Chakra: When this Chakra is blocked, unmotivated mood swings are frequent. You are not able to keep your fears under control. You often find yourself lost in a fantasy world, lost in continuous daydreams. Being the Chakra of our Third Eye, if a veil covers the eye (it blocks the eye), we are not able to see beyond appearances, and we see in a blurred way. For this reason, another symptom of the blockage is the loss of intuition, which makes us close in on ourselves because we can no longer see anything around us, neither material nor spiritual. We tend to worry about any triviality and we are afraid of things that probably will never happen. Nervousness and insomnia are common. So are feelings of apathy, distrust, depression, and a sense of worthlessness. Often accompanying these feelings is the sensation of no longer having feelings because you can't see or recognize them. This is what causes the tendency to live in the world of dreams, so as not to see a surrounding reality that we do not like.

Possible causes of blockage or imbalance: This Chakra is usually blocked when we tend to live in the world of dreams, far away from reality, without ever doing anything to make these dreams come true, and allowing them to remain only fantasies.

Gems of Third Eye Chakra: The main stone of this Chakra is Amethyst. It is in resonance with all purple stones which are powerful in promoting mental processes and concentration. The most popular purple stones are purple zircon, lapis lazuli, calcite, and fluorite.

Associated colors: Indigo and violet

Associated sense: Sixth sense

Associated fragrance: Artemisia, mint, rosemary, lavender, star anise, thyme, and neroli. These are essential oils that stimulate the intellectual and intuitive side, and send messages of a subtle nature.

Associated number: 2

Mantra: AUM

Associated foods: To energize this Chakra you need foods and drinks that stimulate mental energy, such as tea and coffee, for example. Indigo fruits and vegetables, such as eggplant, berries, and grapes, are also good. A good alternative is given by plants with indigo flowers such as rosemary, or juniper, for infusions, and to flavor your dishes.

NOTE: The flow of energy in this Chakra must be balanced and constant because in case of excessive flow you may experience feelings of continuous distraction, and impatience, and you may bring to an access your sense of ambition. When excess of flow in the energy of this Chakra occurs, the person does not take responsibility, tends to exalts his own talents too much, and tends to unload his own faults and errors onto others.

Crown Chakra (7th)

(Sanskrit Name: Sahasrara)

Element: Time and Space

Color: Violet

Position: On the top of the head

Planet: Neptune

Characteristics of the well-balanced Chakra: The seventh Chakra is the center of spirituality, through which we can channel cosmic energy. It gives us purity, helps us to channel our light, makes us creative, and pushes us to constantly improve. It teaches us to trust our inner voice because we have arrived at a very deep knowledge and awareness of ourselves, an almost transcendental knowledge. It makes us skilled observers, able to notice with awareness what is happening around us. The past does not influence us in any way, we have not forgotten it, it simply does not influence us anymore because we have taken responsibility for our mistakes, and we have overcome the traumas. Our thinking is clean and we can recognize our merits as well because we are free from mental impositions. The main purpose of this Chakra is to make us live consciously.

Personal qualities related to this Chakra: Bliss, enlightenment, understanding, universal awareness, and divine wisdom.

Which organs is it associated with? The central nervous system, cerebral cortex, right eye, brain, and skull.

What physical problems is it related to? Among the most frequent physical symptoms are depression, sensitivity to light, and learning difficulties.

What part of the emotional sphere does it influence? This Chakra influences, from the emotional point of view, the understanding both of oneself and of others. In fact, when this Chakra is blocked or unbalanced this understanding is lost, causing the problems discussed below.

Symptoms of a blocked Chakra: When this Chakra is blocked, one tends to be rigid, superficial, unsatisfied, and too attached to material things. High fear of death is very common because it is perceived as the end of everything. We lose sight of the good things in life and feel estranged from everything around us. Often there is a strong attachment to what you have, caused by the thought of not deserving anything else, and for this reason, you constantly belittle yourself.

Possible causes of blockage or imbalance: Usually this Chakra is blocked when we manifest too strong an attachment to the material and earthly world, for example, an excessive attachment to work, home, or people. These excessive sensations of attachment and belonging lead to blocks and imbalances.

Gems of the Crown Chakra: The main stone of this Chakra is the rock crystal (hyaline quartz), which helps to overcome personal problems, and makes us deepen our knowledge of ourselves. This Chakra also resonates with white or transparent stones such as diamond, colorless zircon, iridescent opal, and white agate.

Associated colors: White (because it encloses all colors), transparent and purple

Associated sense: No physical sense

Associated fragrances: Rose, jasmine, sandalwood, lavender, myrrh, and olibanum. These are essential oils with a persistent fragrance that stimulate the connection with the divine and spiritual development.

Associated number: 1000

Associated mantra: OM

Associated Foods: This Chakra benefits from foods and drinks with detoxifying and purifying effects, since it is dealing with less physical energy than the other Chakras. Lotus and lavender are great for balancing and energizing it.

NOTE: Excessive functioning of this Chakra leads to a strong distraction in achieving your goals. If you do not quickly achieve what you want, you tend to give up and this leads you to never achieve anything. Its correct flow in a balanced way is, therefore, fundamental to living a fulfilling and satisfying life.

How to Balance and Heal Your Chakras

In the previous chapter, we looked in detail at each of the 7 main Chakras. At this point, you should have a very clear picture of the sphere of interest of each Chakra and some of the elements that can influence it positively or negatively. For example, now you should be able to recognize what negative behaviors can block the energy flow of a certain Chakra, and also choose what color, stone, or essence can help to heal a certain Chakra, and to make its energy flow correctly. Also, with the knowledge gained, you should be able to identify which ones are your blocked or unbalanced Chakras, so you can start working toward healing them. The section dedicated to the symptoms in each Chakra is the main tool for your diagnosis. If you recognize your current situation in any of the emotional, mental, or physical symptoms described then you know you need to intervene in the Chakra that originates those symptoms. In the next few pages, we will look at the various options available to you to open, unlock, and heal your Chakras. Most options are DIY, for others you might need a little help but you will surely find one or more options suitable for you.

First, however, I would like to bring your attention to an important point: unlocking the Chakras is not permanent. It is an ongoing process. After unlocking a Chakra, a lack of energy may occur, causing a new closure, or an imbalance in the energy flow with the consequent recurrence of related problems. Your goal must, therefore, be to completely avoid blockages and imbalances, and keep the energy flow well and balanced constantly. To do this, you need to take constant care of each one of your Chakras. Always pay attention to symptoms that indicate a lack of energy flow or a potential blockage, try to listen to yourself, and keep an eye and try to notice the signals of your body because this simple step of analysis and awareness will be your first ally in the path for healing Chakras, and to improve your everyday life.

My advice is to create your own regular routine of total care to balance your Chakras so that you can enjoy constant benefits mentally, physically, spiritually, and emotionally. Another piece of advice I would like to give you is to work on all of your Chakras regularly, especially if you are in doubt about which of the 7 Chakras needs the most immediate or major intervention. You may need, especially in the beginning, to work with particular intensity on only one of them at a time, but then you should focus on balancing all 7 to improve your overall mental, physical, spiritual, and emotional health.

There are mainly 7 methods for healing and balancing your Chakras and we will cover them throughout the book. We will see in detail how each technique applies to the different

Chakras, in the meantime, I list below what these methods are, so you can start to get an idea.

Here are the 7 techniques with which you can heal. open and balance your Chakras:

1. Affirmations and Mantra Repetition

2. Meditation

3. Yoga

4. Massage

5. Chromotherapy

6. Crystal Therapy

7. Therapy with Essential Oils

We'll break them all down individually in the next pages and we'll also discuss how, and whether to combine them for maximum results. We'll also discuss the ones you can easily apply on your own and the ones you may need professional support for.

Affirmations and Mantras

I have chosen to begin with Mantras and Affirmations because they are one of the easiest methods to balance the Chakras and, above all, it is a method that you can easily apply on your own, without interfering too much with your everyday habits. Unfortunately, they may not be completely effective on their own, especially in case of imbalances or blockages that are too pronounced, but they help to keep the Chakras in optimal balance if they are practiced regularely (it would be ideal to make them part of a routine, as I suggested before).

My suggestion is to practice this method every day, for a few minutes, focusing each day on a different Chakra. What you have to do is to repeat aloud the affirmation or the specific Mantra of a certain Chakra. No phrase or mantra has an effect on all Chakras at the same time and, for this reason, I suggested that you focus on a Chakra for each day of the week (it is very convenient since there are 7 days and 7 Chakras).

As for the affirmations, I suggest you repeat them out loud while looking in the mirror. Ideally, you should practice these repetitions for a few minutes twice a day, possibly in the morning just after getting up, and in the evening before going to bed. This positive dialogue with yourself brings truly incredible results.

For Mantras, on the other hand, I recommend doing this whenever you have a few free minutes where you can sit in a relaxed pose, with your eyes closed. You will have to pronounce them aloud and the vibrations of those sounds will make you vibrate in tune with the energy of the Chakra you are working on.

In the section where I described the individual Chakras, I listed the Mantra associated with each one but I will list them in the chart below for your convenience. Subsequently, I will list both in detail and in a similar chart the affirmation related to each Chakra, and all my suggestions to optimize the application.

Mantras

Chakra	Mantra
1° Chakra - Root	LAM
2° Chakra - Sacral	VAM
3° Chakra - Solar Plexus	RAM
4° Chakra - Heart	YAM
5° Chakra - Throat	HAM
6° Chakra - Third Eye	AUM
7° Chakra - Crown	OM

Affirmations

I. Root Chakra

The main affirmation related to this Chakra is:

I AM

This affirmation is sufficient to balance the Chakra, but for many, it does not work because they cannot identify with it as it is. Therefore it is often necessary to make the phrase more complete and specific. For example, for many it is useful to say that you are beautiful on a mental or physical level, for others to be safe and have everything you need, for others still to be centered, to be happy, to be in your body and be yourself, and even to be connected to the nature that surrounds you.

"I AM BEAUTIFUL"

"I AM SAFE AND HAVE EVERYTHING I NEED"

"I AM CENTERED AND ROOTED"

"I AM HAPPY TO BE IN MY BODY"

"I AM CONTENT TO BE MYSELF"

"I AM CONNECTED TO NATURE"

II. Sacral Chakra

The main affirmation related to this Chakra is:

I FEEL

This affirmation is about our ability to feel sensations and experience them. As for the previous affirmation, the main sentence "I feel" is sufficient but for many people, it works better to have more complete sentences.

For example:

"I FEEL JOY AND HAPPINESS"

"I FEEL PLEASURE"

"I FEEL CREATIVE"

"I FEEL FULL OF JOY"

"I FEEL SENSUAL AND EMBRACE MY SEXUALITY"

"I FEEL LIKE HONORING MY DESIRES"

"I FEEL PLAYFUL AND SPONTANEOUS"

"I FEEL I DESERVE TO ENJOY LIFE"

"I FEEL HEALTHY"

"I HAVE HEALTHY FEELINGS"

"I FEEL ALIVE AND FACE THE WORLD WITHOUT FEAR"

III. Solar Plexus Chakra

The main affirmation related to this Chakra is:

I DO

You can practice it as it is, or create phrases if you feel more comfortable with them. The affirmations of this Chakra are mainly about action and doing.

For example:

"I ACT WITH COURAGE"

"I CARRY OUT MY TASKS EASILY"

"I HONOR MYSELF"

"I ACT WITH POWER"

"MY POTENTIAL IS UNLIMITED"

"I AM RESPONSIBLE FOR THE ACTIONS IN MY LIFE"

IV. Heart Chakra

The main affirmation related to this Chakra is:

I LOVE

For most people, it is easy to recognize this affirmation as their own and practice it easily as it is. However, it can be enriched by many nuances and you can choose those that best suit you if you prefer them to the main affirmation.

For example:

"I LOVE MYSELF AND OTHERS"

"I AM AN EXPRESSION OF LOVE"

"I DESERVE TO BE LOVED"

"I FORGIVE MYSELF AND OTHERS"

"I FOLLOW THE VOICE OF MY HEART"

"I AM LOVED"

"I ACT WITH LOVE"

"I AM FULL OF LOVE"

V. Throat Chakra

The main affirmation related to this Chakra is:

I SAY

The affirmations linked to this Chakra are associated with speaking and communicating. The main affirmation can be practiced as it is, or you can use the formula "I SPEAK". All for all the previous affirmations, in this case as well you can create richer and more complete affirmations, if they make more sense to you, and make your practice easier.

For example:

"I HEAR AND SPEAK THE TRUTH"

"MY VOICE IS IMPORTANT"

"I SPEAK AND MY WORDS EXPRESS INTEGRITY"

"I SPEAK OPENLY AND HONESTLY AND LIVE AN AUTHENTIC LIFE"

"I RECEIVE AND COMMUNICATE AN IMPORTANT MESSAGE"

"I SPEAK HONEST, TRUE, AND SINCERE WORDS"

VI. Third Eye Chakra

The main affirmation related to this Chakra is:

I SEE

The affirmation of this Chakra is linked to both physical and spiritual sight. The main affirmation is easy to practice for most people and very powerful. However, I list a series of more articulated or complete affirmations, which can give you ideas if you need a full sentence to practice better.

For example:

"I SEE CLEARLY"

"I CAN SEE INTO MYSELF AND OTHERS, AND I AM INTUITIVE"

"I THINK AND I SEE MY THOUGHTS CLEARLY"

"I SEE CLEARLY WHEN I DECIDE AND I TRUST MY DECISIONS"

"I SEE AND THIS EXPANDS MY AWARENESS"

"I BELIEVE IN MY INTUITION AND I TRUST IT"

VII. Crown Chakra

The main affirmation related to this Chakra is:

I UNDERSTAND

The affirmation of this Chakra is linked to the supreme understanding, enlightenment, and comprehension of the all world in its spirituality. The main affirmation can be easily practiced as it is. Even in its simplicity, it contains an incredible strength. It can be varied to "I KNOW" or "I UNDERSTAND" if you feel these phrases are more akin to you. Finally, understanding can be declined in an infinite number of nuances and you may prefer a more articulate statement.

For example:

"I KNOW THAT I AM A DIVINE BEING"

"I KNOW I AM A SPIRITUAL BEING"

"I UNDERSTAND THAT I AM ONE WITH THE WHOLE"

"I KNOW THAT I AM INFINITE AND WITHOUT BOUNDARIES"

"I UNDERSTAND AND I AM AT PEACE"

"I AM OPEN TO UNDERSTANDING AND ENLIGHTENMENT"

Below you can find the resuming chart I promised with the main affirmation of each Chakra. It can be useful to you, just as much as the one I made about the Mantras at the beginning of the chapter. I used to make these little charts for myself when I was just starting my healing journey. I kept a picture of them on my phone and some printed copies in my bag, or in my purse because it took me a little while to learn them by heart. Always having a copy with me helped me a lot in difficult times when I need to practice but I could remember what. You could do this too, it would certainly come in handy and make things a lot easier. When you are starting on a new habit, the easier the better, trust me on this.

Chakra	Mantra
1° Chakra - Root	I AM
2° Chakra - Sacral	I FEEL
3° Chakra - Solar Plexus	I DO
4° Chakra - Heart	I LOVE
5° Chakra - Throat	I SAY
6° Chakra - Third Eye	I SEE
7° Chakra - Crown	I UNDERSTAND

Meditation

Meditation helps us to awaken the energy of our body and, for this reason, is an excellent cure for our closed, blocked, or unbalanced Chakras. Meditation, like Mantras and affirmations, is a method that you can apply with total autonomy. This makes it very useful and valuable because you can practice it whenever you want and feel the need for it. You don't depend on the help of others to practice it and that's great because, if you live on a busy schedule, you can just arrange the opportunity to practice during a coffee or lunch break.

Many people are afraid of the idea of meditating because they believe they are not able to do it. In truth, it's very easy! To start meditating you just need to let your thoughts free to flow or hold one thought and let all the others flow away from your head. Meditating for the Chakras does not require particularly high or transcendental meditation techniques, just simple visualization exercises, appropriate music, and breathing correctly.

So, meditating for the Chakras is really simple and you can refine your technique with repetition and practice. Also, the more time you dedicate to this activity, the greater the results you will get. You can start by dedicating just a few minutes a day to meditation to begin to see the first positive changes and improvements. As you invest more time in the activity of meditation you will be able to see bigger and better results.

You can meditate on a single Chakra, or you can work on all of them simultaneously, according to your needs and requirements. This makes this practice even greater because it allows you to take care of all your Chakras at one time.

You could, or rather you should create a meditation corner. You should choose a quiet place just for yourself, possibly in your house. You should decorate your meditation space with cushions and mats to be comfortable, and surround yourself with objects, colors, stones, and essences to further stimulate your Chakras. (We will talk more about this further stimulation of your Chakras later).

Now let's look at the strongest but simplest meditation techniques that you can start applying immediately to heal, unblock, and balance your Chakras.

Color Meditation

The color meditation is the simplest Chakra meditation. Even if it is so simple it has a great impact on your Chakras' health.

Let's see how to practice it step-by-step.

1. First of all, you will need to find a quiet place where you feel comfortable or simply go to your meditation corner if you have organized one. You will have to sit in a comfortable position and I recommend wearing comfortable clothes to be as comfortable as possible. It would be ideal to have a straight back so that all the Chakras are aligned during the meditation.

2. Now close your eyes. Breath with your nose. Concentrate on your breathing for a few minutes and take deep breaths in a single air flux. Inhale for about 4 seconds and exhale all the air you let in taking exactly the same amount of time, 4 seconds. Keep breathing in this way during all the practice.

3. Starting from the lowest Chakra, visualize the color of that Chakra, feel pervaded by the energy of that color,

and keep this thought and this sensation for at least 4 minutes, during which the color inside you should become brighter and brighter.

4. Use your breath to give a rhythm to your meditation, every time you inspire the color pervades you more and becomes more intense and brilliant.

5. After at least 4 minutes you can move on to the next color, and repeat the sequence from step 3 until you have covered the entire color spectrum of your 7 Chakras. When you are finished, wait a few seconds then slowly open your eyes.

You can practice this meditation in different ways:

- You can go through all 7 Chakra colors. This is useful if you are working on maintaining the balance of all the Chakras.

- You can work on one Chakra at a time. If you feel a particular pleasure in working on one color, it may be that that particular color needs more attention, so you could devote yourself only to it, and stay on it for the whole meditation time. The same if you already know you have to work on a particular Chakra, you will devote the entire meditation to its color.

- If you only have small spaces of time to dedicate to meditation, that's fine too. It would be ideal to be able to do at least 5 minutes at a time, several times a day if you can. Choose, according to your needs, whether to practice a different color at each session or to focus on the same color each time.

- I summarized, in the chart below, the color of each Chakra for your convenience, in case you haven't memorized them yet. I already explained the bests you can do with these charts.

Chakra	Color
1º Chakra - Root	RED
2º Chakra - Sacral	ORANGE
3º Chakra - Solar Plexus	YELLOW
4º Chakra - Heart	GREEN
5º Chakra - Throat	LIGHT BLUE
6º Chakra - Third Eye	INDIGO
7º Chakra - Crown	VIOLET

The 7 Chakras' Meditation

The 7 Chakras' meditation is a little more articulated than the previous one and is extremely powerful. Let's see together, step-by-step, how to practice it in the most correct and effective way:

1. You will need to find a quiet place where you feel comfortable or simply go to your meditation corner. You will need to sit in a comfortable position and I recommend wearing comfortable clothes to be as comfortable as possible and in a general condition of easiness. It would be ideal to sit with a straight back so that all the Chakras are aligned during the meditation. Close your eyes.

2. Breath with your nose. Concentrate on your breathing for a few minutes and take deep breaths in a single air flux. Inhale for about 4 seconds and exhale all the air you let in taking exactly the same amount of time, 4 seconds. Keep breathing in this way during all the practice.

3. After about a minute or two of concentrating on breathing, you should begin to focus on every part of your body, starting from your head down to your feet. You will need to relax each part of your body that you focus on. Try to see in your mind's eye every single muscle that relaxes as you focus on it: your forehead

flattening, your lips stretching, your neck releasing the tension, and so on down to your toes. This is important because you don't want to be too tense or stiff in your sitting position.

4. Now let's move on to breathing. You will have to focus your attention on your breathing: inhale and exhale, in and out. You don't have to force it in any way, just keep focusing your attention on it and you will see that it will slowly become deeper and deeper and more regular. While you are putting air into your lungs, try to visualize it. Try to see the air that enters your lungs, spreads through the blood, enters the muscles, and every cell in your body. When you let the air out, visualize the air coming out of your body taking with it all the toxins and garbage that clog your body. Remember always to breathe through your nose so that fewer impurities enter your body.

5. When you feel your breath proceeding naturally deeply and regularly, you should turn your concentration to your heartbeat. Visualize your heart beating and, at each pulse, moves your blood to reach every part of your body. When the blood reaches every part of your body all those parts enter in harmony and communication with each other. Travel with your blood, reach every part of your

body and feel this wonderful living organism full of strength and energy. Each breath makes your heart beat and brings your body to life.

6. Now imagine that with each breath you take, you let energy into your body, an energy that flows into you along with the air and pervades you with a life force. Create a clear image in your mind. See this energy flowing into your body, see your body absorbing the energy, and becoming stronger. It is a gradual process, with each breath your body becomes stronger and more enlightened by this wonderful energy until your body will glow with a clear and brilliant halo. Build a clear picture of this halo in your mind.

7. Now, you have to channel this energy into each Chakra. As always, you will have to start from the lowest Chakra, the Root, and gradually move upward until you reach the Crown. You will have to visualize your Chakra as a small luminous sphere that rotates clockwise. With each breath, the sphere receives energy and becomes stronger and brighter. You must repeat this visualization for each Chakra until the one you are focused on is full of vital energy. It takes time and some Chakras will take longer than others. When a Chakra takes longer to feel full of energy is because that particular Chakra needs more care

than another. Your mind knows this and guides you through the healing process. In this phase, it is important to move in an orderly way from the bottom to the top without haste, dedicating to each Chakra the time it needs. This is because each Chakra is connected to the one above it and by practicing in the correct we can maintain a perfect balance.

8. Once you have concluded the visualization process for each of the 7 Chakras, take a few seconds, and then slowly open your eyes. Before getting up, I suggest you take a few minutes to try to understand how you feel physically, mentally, spiritually, and emotionally. This moment of analysis is very important both because you will enjoy the pleasant sensations that meditation leaves you and because it will serve as a parameter. Each time you stop to analyze your meditation, you will find that you feel better than the previous time in at least one of the four areas but more often in all four at the same time. You'll feel better physically, mentally, spiritually, and emotionally.

This meditation, being a bit more structured, takes at least half an hour to practice. Some speak of completing it in a quarter of an hour, I personally never managed to complete it in such a short time. My advice is not to rush it and if you already know that you don't have at least thirty minutes, you could fall back on the color meditation which is a good faster option.

Meditating on a single Chakra

It is also possible to concentrate the meditation on a single Chakra if instead of creating a general balance we need to quickly heal a particularly suffering Chakra.

The preparation is the same as described in steps 1 through 6 of the "7 Chakras' Meditation". In step 7, instead of gradually going through all 7 Chakras from bottom to top, you will concentrate only and exclusively on the Chakra you need to quickly heal.

You will have to channel the energy generated in the first 6 steps into the Chakra you are working on. All your concentration will have to be on it. Visualize your small luminous sphere that rotates clockwise, with each breath the sphere receives energy and becomes stronger and brighter. You will have to dedicate to this Chakra all the time it needs and repeat the process daily until you feel you have healed it.

In this regard, never skip the last step, the one of analysis, and understanding because only through it you can understand how you feel physically, mentally, spiritually, and emotionally after each meditation.

The average time required by the meditation on a single Chakra is at least 10-15 minutes, a time easier to carve out than the 30 minutes of the complete 7 Chakras' meditation. One thing that over time I have found very useful is to practice the complete sequence of the 7 Chakras' meditation once a week and then practice the single Chakra meditation once a day for the next 7 days, addressing the Chakras in order from lowest to highest. This is a suggestion for those with limited time, but I think it will come in handy as you build your Chakras' healing routine. I have learned from personal experience that you need to find the best way to fit these important moments into your hectic daily life, and organizing a routine that takes into account the time you have available daily is essential. If you don't create your own Chakra healing routine, you won't benefit from it in the end, and this book will have been nothing more than a pleasant read.

By consistently practicing Chakras' meditation, in any of its variations, you will see incredible results in your daily life, on all levels: in your professional life, in your personal and emotional life, and even in your health. You will gain an inner wholeness and lucidity that will give you noticeable results on a physical, mental, spiritual, and emotional level.

Earth's Meditation

A meditation that has always made me feel very good when I needed to gain energy to balance my Chakras is the one called "Earth's meditation".

This form of meditation consists exactly of the first 6 steps of the 7 Chakras' meditation with two fundamental differences. First, it should not be practiced indoors but outdoors, sitting in close contact with Mother Earth (hence its name). So, eyes closed, back straight, but sitting in a quiet corner in the middle of nature: in a park, a forest, near a stream, on the shore of a lake, or any other place of natural wonder where you feel good and comfortable.

Second, when you have accumulated all the energy through the 6 steps, you will not need to focus on the Chakras, but you will need to stay focused on the life force that is coming to you from nature and Mother Earth. You will have to continue to focus on your breathing, on this life force that grows inside you, pervades you every time you inhale, and expels negative energy and toxins every time you exhale.

It is impossible to estimate a time for this meditation because you merge so much with the nature around you that you could practice it for hours without noticing the passage of time. Of course, it is not so easy to practice it because it is not easy to find quiet corners of unspoiled nature unless you are lucky enough to live in the countryside outside the city.

I invite you, however, to seek out these corners and these moments from time to time because the well-being that this meditation can give you is impossible to describe in words. For me, it has always been a bit like recharging my personal batteries with energy that my Chakras will channel and make flow.

Again, I invite you not to forget point 8. Open your eyes when you have finished your meditation, but before you get up, take all the time you need to understand how you feel physically, mentally, spiritually, and emotionally, and to fully enjoy that wonderful feeling of well-being that I am sure will pervade you.

In the beginning, it will probably feel a little strange to meditate on your Chakras, especially if you have never meditated before in your life but with time and practice it will become as natural as breathing and you won't be able to do without because it will make you feel infinitely good on every level.

Tricks for Chakra Meditation

There are small elements that you can implement during your meditation to favor the energy of a Chakra rather than another, or even make the energy of individual Chakras more effective. Let's see what they are for every single Chakra and how to use them to your advantage:

- **1st Chakra:** To release tension and get even better results when meditating for this Chakra, the ideal would be to meditate while sitting on the ground. Not necessarily outdoors, although that would be even better. This is because it is the Root Chakra, the root that sinks into Mother Earth and the earth is its element.

- **2nd Chakra:** The Sacral Chakra is strongly linked to the element of water. If you meditate for this Chakra you could put the sound of waves, flowing, or gurgling water in the background to make the meditation more powerful. You could also meditate sitting in the bathtub, partially immersed in the water.

- **3rd Chakra:** If you meditate for the Solar Plexus Chakra, the fundamental element to make the meditation more effective is silence. It is characteristic of this Chakra to maintain attention, calm, and silence. Using these three elements during your meditation is very useful for the 3rd

Chakra. Silence itself could be a form of meditation for the health of this Chakra.

- **4th Chakra:** The element of the heart Chakra is air and breathing is the fundamental element if you meditate for this Chakra. You have learned in this chapter the importance of breathing during meditation, importance that becomes even greater when you meditate for the fourth Chakra.

- **5th Chakra:** For the Throat Chakra, words are a magical instrument whose vibrations put us in tune with the universe. To make the meditation for this Chakra more intense, you could repeat a mantra while meditating, or chant.

- **6th Chakra:** The last two Chakras are much more connected to spirituality, so to favor them during meditation you will have to do things less related to the physical world. To better meditate on the Third Eye Chakra you will have to free your mind from the thoughts that continue to crowd it and try to acquire a clearer inner vision.

- **7th Chakra:** To intensify the meditation for the Crown Chakra you will have to expand your connection with the universal energy and focus deeply on your spirituality and on the awareness that you are a spiritual being in a physical body.

Yoga

At this point, we can safely say that the Chakras are a fundamental tool to take care of to maintain ourselves and our bodies in good health at all levels. From this point of view, we can say that yoga is a kind of architect that allows us to implement this project of taking care of ourselves. There are specific positions that allow us to balance or unlock every Chakra.

Although it is a very effective method, you may not be able to use it in total autonomy. If you have had previous experience with yoga and have learned the fundamentals you won't experience any problems. If, however, you are completely new to this discipline, it would be ideal to take a few lessons with an experienced teacher to learn the basics that will allow you to proceed on your own. There are also many good and useful online yoga academies. They give you the chance to attend yoga classes according to your schedule. It is very important to have these basics because mistakes in practice or posture could lead to physical damage, easily avoidable with the advice of an expert. If, however, you already know the basics, many positions can help you unlock your Chakras. Let's see 7 of them, one for each Chakra:

1st Chakra - Root: *Position Of The Tree* (Vrksasana)

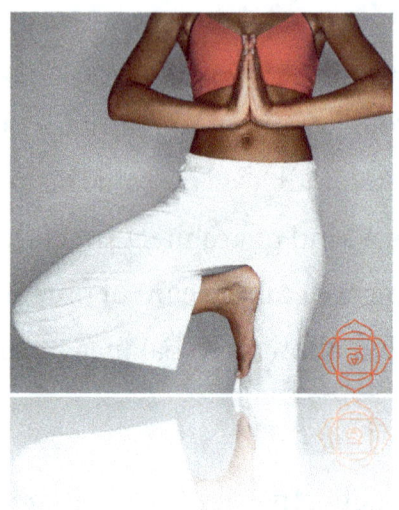

2nd Chakra - Sacral: *Position Of The Goddess* (Deviasana)

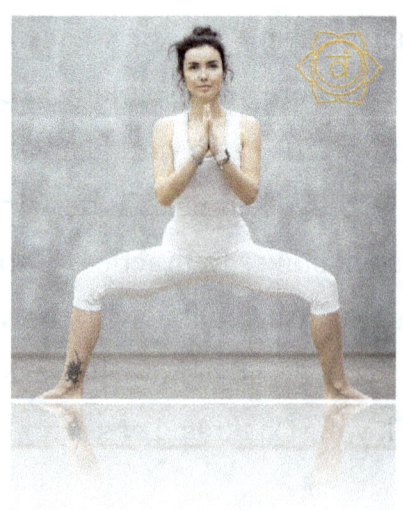

3rd Chakra - Solar Plexus: <u>*Position Of The Boat*</u>
(Navasana)

4th Chakra - Heart: <u>*Position Of The Camel*</u> *(Ustrasana)*

5th Chakra - Throat: <u>Position Of The Candle With Support</u> (Salamba Sarvangasana)

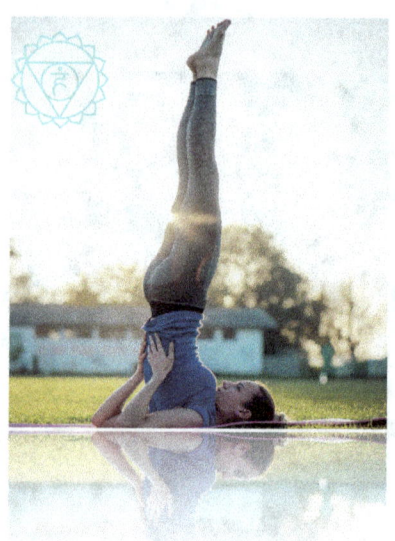

6th Chakra - Third Eye: <u>Comfortable Position</u> (Sukhasana)

7th Chakra - Crown: <u>Corpse Position</u> (Savasana)

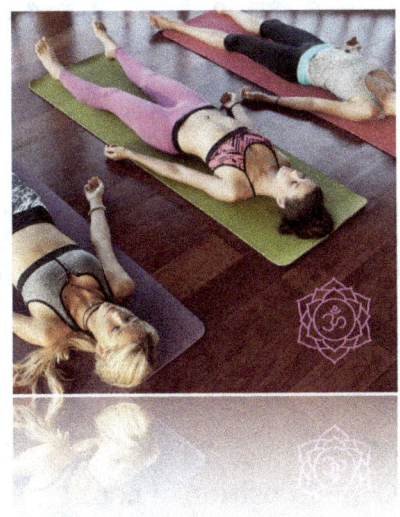

You can do the sequence in full and in order, as always from the bottom Chakra up, or you can focus on the Chakra you are working on. You can also work on two or three Chakras only. In this case, pick the yoga poses of each Chakra you are working on to build your yoga sequence, your choice depends on the areas of your life you are focusing on that require healing.

If during your practice you experience a sense of restlessness that you cannot easily calm or control my advice is to hold the position(s) you are practicing longer. This will help you to be more present and grounded, and to eliminate the sense of restlessness.

Breathing is very important when practicing yoga, just as much as when practicing meditation. You can use the same kind of breathing technique we discussed in the chapter about meditation.

Breath with your nose. Inhale and exhale from a single flux of air. Take 4 seconds every time you inhale and 4 seconds when you exhale. Take long, relaxed, and deep breaths. Remember to breathe even when you are holding a position. To help me with this, I count the breaths for each position I hold. For example, when I hold the "Camel Position" I count 3 complete sequences of breathing before changing position. My exceptions are Sukhasana e Savasana. In Sukhasana I only concentrate on breathing properly, in Savasana I let my body totally relax and I let my breath run freely according to my relaxed condition.

Just so you know, the name of this breathing technique is "Ujjayi Breathing" ("The Winning Breath") and it has one more main characteristic apart from the ones already described. When breathing, you should try to close a little the top part of your throat so that the air stays longer in the top part of your breathing system. In this way, air maintains a longer contact with your mucous membrane rich in blood, which makes the air you breathe a lot warmer, giving your body a relaxed feeling.

Massages

If you have experienced a massage at least once in your life, you know how beneficial it is for your body, your mind, and your spirit. When you are massaged you feel all the tension in your body melt away, stress leaves you, and you feel in a delightful state of absolute grace for a few days after.

This wonderful practice can be used to help your Chakras, to open them up, and to keep them in balance. Not all Chakras need the same type of massage, in fact, the type of massage varies depending on the Chakra you want to work on and its location.

To get the most out of this practice my advice is to ask an expert, so you can let yourself go completely and enjoy the massage in total relaxation. It is however possible to stimulate some areas of your body with a DIY massage that helps to heal your Chakras.

In the following pages, we will see what area to massage and how so that you can stimulate every Chakra on your own. Still, I suggest you go to an expert whenever possible to fully enjoy this wonderful experience. If you are not used to massaging, at first this practice may make you feel a little awkward. Don't worry, all you need is a little practice, and it will soon become a natural gesture that will amaze you with its simplicity, effectiveness, and great results.

The correct way to massage yourself to stimulate and activate your Chakras' energy is with a few simple slow circular movements in a clockwise direction. When you begin to feel comfortable with those movements and the massage, you can try speeding up the rhythm or increasing the pressure. Find the combination that gives you the most pleasant sensation in each part of your body and practice it for 5 to 10 minutes, daily.

As for the methods I described in the previous chapters, you can practice the massage in two ways. You can go through all your Chakras from the bottom one to the top one or you can work with one in particular at a time. If you have little time to dedicate to this practice but you want to work on all the Chakras, you can focus on one single Chakra per day. If you choose this option, remember to always massage your Chakras' in order starting from the bottom and going upward. For example, start on Monday massaging your body to stimulate energy in the Root Chakra, on Tuesday to stimulate the Sacral Chakra, and so on with the rest of the days of the week.

For massage, just like I suggested for meditation, you should create a quiet corner where you can retreat and practice. Peace, silence, and tranquility will help you to put your body in a relaxed state that will make the massage easier and more effective.

To make your hands flow better on your skin, essential oils are an excellent solution. We will see in the dedicated chapter how you can choose oils whose essence and fragrance help the opening and stimulation of the Chakra you are working on healing.

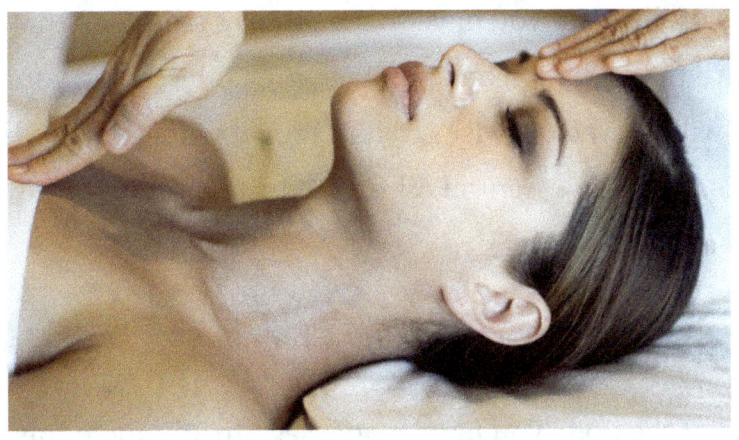

Let's look at the areas to massage for each Chakra:

I. The Root Chakra

The parts of the body you have to massage to stimulate this Chakra are the buttocks, legs, and feet. Dedicate a pleasant massage to this area of your body and let the feeling of well-being radiate throughout your body.

II. The Sacral Chakra

The parts of the body you have to massage to stimulate this Chakra are the area below the navel, the hip area, the lumbar muscles, and the base of the back.

III. The Solar Plexus Chakra

The parts of the body you have to massage to stimulate this Chakra are the abdomen and stomach area. Massaging your stomach with slow clockwise circular movements and hands lightly greased with essential oil will activate an important energy center for your body.

IV. The Heart Chakra

The parts of the body you have to massage to stimulate this Chakra are the chest, shoulders, the beginning of the arm, and the back of the torso. Some areas are difficult to reach, so, do what you can without tugging or straining, and try to keep your muscles relaxed as much as possible. Start with slow circles on the chest, rising just as slowly to the shoulders, then move to the beginning of the arms, and when you move to the back of the torso reach as far as you can without strain or tension.

V. The Throat Chakra

The parts of the body you have to massage to stimulate this Chakra go from the base of the neck, down to the shoulders, going all the way through the neck. Start with light and slow circular rubs from the hairline of the head towards the neck, go down along the back of the neck, and then slowly focus on the muscles that connect the neck to the shoulders. Continue until you feel the desired effect of the tension easing.

VI. The Third Eye Chakra

To stimulate this Chakra we focus on massaging the area of the face, always with slow circular movements. Begin with the temples, forehead, cheeks, cheekbones, and then the jaws. I recommend that you perform this massage with your eyes closed, trying to relax as much as possible. This will help you to better enjoy the feeling of opening your third eye.

VII. The Crown Chakra

This Chakra is stimulated by massaging the head area from the hairline to the entire scalp area. When practiced well and regularly, this massage allows you to enjoy a wonderful feeling of pressure easing, and energy flowing.

A consistent practice of massage will be extremely beneficial in rebalancing and healing your chakras, and you will feel increasingly filled with a new positive and beneficial energy that flows through your body.

Chromotherapy

Chromotherapy is treating the Chakras with the colors of the rainbow.

Our body reacts to colors because each color is a different vibration of energy. According to Ayurvedic medicine, since our body reacts to colors on a physical, emotional, spiritual, and mental level, the 7 colors of the rainbow can rebalance the energy centers of our body, your 7 main Chakras. The principle behind this idea is that life is color and color is life, as opposed to the darkness and gloom of death.

The 7 colors of the rainbow, therefore, restore the balance of our energy centers and influence their health daily. This daily influence manifests itself in an infinite number of ways since most of the objects that surround us are colored. The food you eat, the colors of the clothes you wear, and the colors of the environment in which you live or work influence your Chakras and your energy in every single moment of your life. The influence can be positive or negative. Think about a horrible working place, decorated with colors that make you feel upset or uncomfortable, that's definitely a negative way to use the power of colors in your life. On the other hand, if you use this power with consciousness and a positive purpose, it can bring enormous benefits to the energy flow of your Chakras.

Reflecting light through a prism, we obtain the 7 colors of the rainbow. Those colors show themselves to our eyes in a sequence exactly equivalent to the Chakras' colors, ordered from first to last Chakra.

The highest color of the prism corresponds to the first Chakra, the one with the lowest position on the spine. Going down in the colors' sequence of the prism, we go up with the position of the Chakras along the spine.

So:

First Chakra: *Mūlādhāracakra* = Red

Second Chakra: *Svādhisthānacakra* = Orange

Third Chakra: *Manipura* = Yellow

Fourth Chakra: *Anahata* = Green

Fifth Chakra: *Vishudda* = Blue

Sixth Chakra: *Ajna* = Indigo Blue

Seventh Chakra: *Sahasrara* = Violet

Since each Chakra is represented by a different color and since there are so many ways to give color to your life, you can take care of each Chakra very easily. Chromotherapy is another method that you can use in total autonomy, you don't need any help to apply it, you just need to memorize the color associated with each Chakra. The enormous advantage of this method is that it takes no time at all, you only need to do is to choose carefully and consciously the colors that fill your life.

The three areas where you can use chromotherapy most effectively are your clothing, the food you eat, and your surroundings. For example, if you are working on the Sacral Chakra, you could wear a bright orange t-shirt, eat a juicy orange, and lay a bright orange bedspread on your bed.

Chromotherapy is a great way to work on multiple Chakras and also a quick way to intervene on a single one if you feel a momentary imbalance. When you get dressed in the morning you should choose at least one piece of clothing in the color of the Chakra you feel needs energizing. You should do the same with food, including in your food plan some food in harmony with the color of the Chakra to be harmonized.

As for the surrounding environment, since you can not change furniture too frequently, my advice is to create "spaces" dedicated to each one of the 7 colors in your house and in your working place. Then, you will only need to spend some time in a certain space when you feel the need to work on one color rather than another one. For example, you may need to spend 15 minutes on your "Red Space" because, at some point in your day, you don't feel as rooted in the moment as you should be.

One area that I recommend you devote a lot of attention to is your meditation corner. I have chosen to have in mine all the 7 colors represented in equivalent parts and then, when I feel the need for the predominance of the color of a certain Chakra, I temporarily add some object or decoration to make that color prevail over the others. Maybe I add a pillow, some flowers, a yoga mat, a stone, or a crystal that I then move and replace when I need to balance another Chakra associated with another color.

This last paragraph also introduced an important and interesting concept. Techniques for healing your Chakras often cross over, overlap, and support each other. For example, in your meditation corner in addition to the benefits of meditation, you will enjoy the benefits of chromotherapy, crystals, gemstones, and essential oils.

The care of the Chakras through colors is still a very effective technique, even alone, to find the balance of your Chakras and heal eventual blocks in the fluxing of energy.

Crystal Therapy

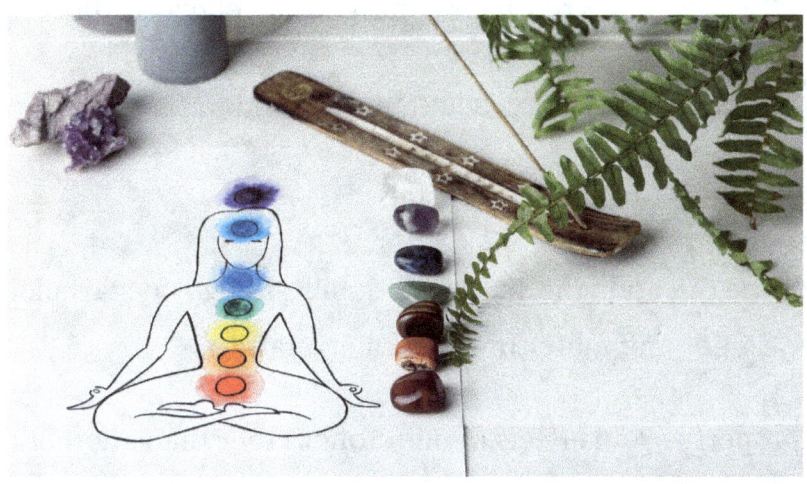

Crystal therapy allows us to use the power of stones, crystals, and minerals to restore the energetic balance of our Chakras, open them and unblock their energy flow if blocked. This method can be easily used in total independence.

To each specific Chakra corresponds a group of specific stones, as we have seen in the descriptive section of the 7 Chakras. The association between stone and Chakra occurs through color. The prevailing tonality of a Chakra is in resonance with the color of the stone. I summarized the color correspondence briefly below for your convenience. However, you can easily go back to the chapter titled "The 7 Main Chakras" to get more details on color correspondence, names of adequate gems, and crystals.

- For the 1st Chakra red, brown, and black crystals

- For the 2nd and 3rd Chakra orange and yellow crystals

- For the 4th Chakra green and pink crystals

- For the 5th Chakra blue crystals

- For the 6th and 7th Chakras dark blue-indigo crystals plus all the lighter and more transparent crystals.

The properties and effects of one stone rather than another one are subjected to its chemical and physical characteristics, as well as its color. For example, a piece of quartz and a piece of calcite of the same color will have different applications. The stones "preferred" by crystal therapy are, as you can deduce from the very name of this practice, quartz crystals. The crystal, in fact, has a high ability to absorb energy and activate the energy spectrum of a person. Crystals also stimulate intuition and awaken insight, helping us to nurture our spirituality, and supporting us in introspection, that is, helping us in our process of acquiring awareness.

There are many methods of using the power of stones to open, unlock and balance your Chakras. In the next pages, I will share with you the most important, useful, and easy to use.

Jewelry

There are jewelry pieces such as bracelets or necklaces that have different spherical stones strung in a sequence, just like the image below. They resonate with each one of the 7 Chakras.

Wearing this jewelry regularly is a first step in harnessing the power of the stones to your advantage. This is nothing particularly expensive, it is jewelry made from hard stones and crystals, not precious stones. The shape of the stones is also not random, they are spherical to recall the shape and etymology of the Chakras. There are also variations of these jewels made with a single stone to work on a specific Chakra.

Corresponding Position Between Stone and Chakra

You'll need a set of stones, small enough in size, to perform this practice. You can easily find on sale in many shops ready-made kits containing a stone for each Chakra. I recommend, however, to go to a specialized store, if you have the opportunity, and personally choose a stone suitable to you for each Chakra. Take several stones in your hands, one at a time, and when you take the right one for you, you will feel it, because you will recognize the vibrations it is sending you.

When you have your 7 stones, using them will be very easy. You will need to lie down in a quiet and peaceful place, your meditation corner will be perfect if you have one set up. Then you will have to place each stone directly on your skin, in correspondence with the position in your body of the equivalent Chakra.

When the crystals are positioned you will have to close your eyes, concentrate on breathing, and visualize the energy of the stone placed on the first Chakra. The stone will do all the work, you just need to visualize for a few minutes, and then move on to the next stone and the next Chakra. You will have to proceed in order until you reach the Crown. You should lie there for at least 20 minutes, feeling the energy penetrating your body, and how the energy of each stone is channeled into its respective Chakra. In these 20 minutes, you should not move, you should not speak and you should let your thoughts be free to flow in your mind. Make sure that your breathing is steady and deep. Breathe through your nose. You should find this easy enough since you learned these basics in the chapter on meditation. Once you are done, take a few minutes before opening your eyes, during such time analyze how you feel, and enjoy the energy that is flowing through your body. Before you stand up again you will need to remove the stones. The removal should be in the opposite direction of placement, so you will need to start from the Crown and work your way down to the Root. (You may also choose to get help during the placement and removal if you have a trusted person who can help you, the important thing is that placement and removal are done in the correct order).

As in other practices, you can also practice this exercise on a single Chakra. You will use the single stone positioned on the Chakra concerned, in direct contact with your skin, and proceed with breathing and visualization, as explained in the previous lines.

In the following chart you will find an example of a stone for each Chakra and where to place it for a correct correspondence with its related Chakra:

Chakra	Crystal or Gem	Body Position
1° Chakra	Red Dispore	Groin
2° Chakra	Amber	Pelvis
3° Chakra	Citrin Quartz	Just above the navel
4° Chakra	Jade	Above the heart
5° Chakra	Aquamarine	On the throat
6° Chakra	Amethyst	On the forehead
7° Chakra	Hyaline Quartz	Press it on the top of your head, then place it on the surface where you are lying at the top of your head

Other Uses of Stones

There are many other options for using the energy and power of stones, gems, and crystals to your advantage. Since you can choose from a variety of sizes, there are so many uses to which they lend themselves.

For example, if you choose rather small pieces you could always carry one with you in your pocket and enjoy its energy constantly. Just reach into your pocket and squeeze your stone for an energy booster anytime you feel it's needed.

If you move frequently for work, you could keep one in your car to energize the environment in which you will be moving around. If you move by other means, you could put one in your bag or suitcase to carry the energy with you and feel its presence even when you are traveling.

As you can see, there are many ideas and, for sure, you will come up with others dictated by the very energy of the stones that will communicate with you. For example, I always keep one under the pillow I sleep with. I pick a different crystal every week and I change it on a color rotation.

It is also useful to surround yourself with stones by using them to decorate your surroundings. For this option, it is usually better to choose larger stones. Place one for each Chakra at different points of the house so that their energy surrounds you. Having them around will make you feel better and you will find yourself walking around the house with a smile on your face. I recommend this decorative method in your meditation corner as well. Place a stone for each Chakra to decorate your corner, enrich the energy already present, and give more effectiveness to all the activities that you will do in that space. As I mentioned before, here are the various healing methods that intertwine with each other to give you greater results and an overall sensation of well-being.

Programming Your Stones

It is possible to program stones and crystals to get even more benefits from them. Programming a stone can help you heal an emotional wound, relieve an unpleasant physical sensation, help you meditate, or support you in a time of need. You can also simply program it to let you know if it needs to be purified or recharged with new energy.

Programming a crystal is very simple, just communicate with it. You will need to sit in a quiet and peaceful place where you feel comfortable, like your meditation corner, for example. You will have to close your eyes, enclose the stone inside your hand, feel it, and then start talking to it. The stone will hear you and, within a short time, you will receive your responses in the form of insights. Examples of stones' programming are, "Please, can you give me support today?"; "Please, can you tell me when you need to be purified or recharged?"; "Please, can you tell me what is the right choice to heal from my disappointment in love?". You can program your gems, stones, and crystals with this method for whatever need you might have.

Dialogue with your stones is very important and will make a difference in the results. You must put your heart into it and speak with intentionality. If you do it skeptically or just for the sake of doing it, it won't work. Listen to your heart and it will help you build an effective dialogue between you and your stone. Remember to choose the correct stone, choose one that corresponds to the Chakra that deals with the area of your request. For example, if your request is connected to emotions you need to pick a gem or a crystal in resonance with the Heart Chakra. If it is a request based on material things you need to pick a gemstone or a crystal in resonance with the Root Chakra.

Once you have programmed your stone, as your days go by, you will feel impulses, intuitions, and sensations that your stone will send you in response. For example, it will come to your mind to purify or recharge your stone, you will feel a sensation of support in the moment of need, or you will feel you must go to a certain place, where you will meet someone who, in time, will make you forget your disappointment of love.

Take a few minutes to program your stones and crystals. They will become your greatest allies in achieving mental, emotional, spiritual, and physical well-being. Trust me, you will feel like you own a real magical amulet.

Purifying Your Stones

Stones and crystals not only take energy from us, but also from our surroundings. This means that if you live in cities or highly populated places your crystals and stones will need to be cleansed from time to time of low frequency or unpleasant energies assimilated into your surroundings.

There are three main methods for purifying stones:

1. WATER: This first method is the simplest, but is ineffective on some particular stones. Use your dialogue with the stone to see if the cleaning is successful, or, if in doubt, use the third method which is the most effective. Simply place the stone under running water and, as you do so, visualize the unpleasant energy draining from the stone, and running away with the water.

2. WATER AND SALT: Again, this technique is not suitable for all stones because, although salt is a great purifier, it may damage some of the more polished or shiny stones. However, if you are certain that your stone is compatible with this method, simply soak it overnight in a glass of water and salt, then rinse it under running water the next morning. If in doubt about this method, I recommend using the third method, since it is the safest and most reliable.

3. INCENSE: This is the best and most effective method and, moreover, is good for all stones. Just light a natural incense and pass the stone in its smoke for about 30 seconds. As you do so, you should visualize the unpleasant energy that leaves your stone. You can also ask aloud as you perform the purification ritual, "Please cleanse this stone of any unpleasant energy, thank you!"

Just as with programming, the intentionality of the gesture is fundamental. Don't do it mechanically, just for the sake of doing it, but do it with the intention of purifying your crystals to get the maximum benefit from them. This will make a huge difference to the effectiveness of your purification rituals.

Recharging Your Stones

Recharging your stones periodically with beneficial energy is of fundamental importance because they will then share this energy with you.

There are three main methods for recharging stones and crystals with beneficial energy:

1. THE SUN: The best sunlight to energize your stones is at dawn. Expose the stones in a place where they can get direct sunlight in the early morning. A couple of hours will be sufficient. Ideally, this should be from 6 to 8 a.m., in winter even up to 9 a.m. Remember to remove your stones and crystals from the sun when the light is particularly intense, to avoid damaging them. A timer or an alarm clock will be useful as a reminder.

2. THE MOON: To energize your stones through the moonlight, you'll need a full moon night. Simply display your stones and crystals somewhere in the house near a window where they can enjoy the benefits of the full moon's light. You will need to remove the stones from where you placed them before sunrise before the sunlight hits them in full.

3. THE EARTH: To use the earth's energy on your stones, trees are perfect, but a potted plant will also do. You will need to place the stones on the earth at the foot of the tree or in the pot of your plant. If the sun is beating down at the location you've chosen, you'll need to place your stones in a small hole dug in the earth, and cover them. You can wrap them in a bit of paper to prevent them from getting dirty. It will only take a few hours to energize your stones with soil, but you can also leave them for a few days in total safety.

Essential Oils Therapy

When I discussed the characteristics of every single Chakra, I also described the scents connected to each of them. The scents that we associate with each Chakra are essential oils from plants that can be used in many simple ways to have results similar to chromotherapy and crystal therapy.

Each essential oil has its own Chakra and there are many options for using these oils. The simplest method is to use a "burner" that will spread the chosen fragrance throughout your home or other surroundings. This practice is called aromatherapy. Just pour a few drops of oil into the water of your burner, turn on the flame underneath, and immediately the fragrance will begin to spread in the air (the method described is that of a classic burner, but there are many varieties and each comes with instructions if should follow carefully).

This method is great to practice in your meditation corner because it can easily be combined with other healing techniques to make them even more effective. For example, if you are meditating for a particular Chakra, sprinkling the aroma of the oil associated with it will make your meditation much deeper and more effective.

Another use of essential oils extremely effective to unlock and balance your Chakras is to use them during massages directly on your skin. Essential oils facilitate the massage by making your hands glide better. To perform the massage you must mix a few drops of the essential oil chosen to treat your Chakra with a neutral oil specifically for massage (for example, jojoba oil). It is important to treat only one Chakra at a time with this method, making the massage with extreme delicacy, and dedicating to the massage all the time necessary to open, unblock the energy, and put it back into circulation.

In one of the previous paragraphs, you learned how and which areas to massage to open, unblock, and balance a Chakra. By combining the massage with the essential oil corresponding to that Chakra, you can double the effectiveness of your massage, and the energy released. If you like, without exaggerating, you can also diffuse in the environment the same fragrance you are using for the massage, involving more senses in the unlocking and balancing of your energies.

Let's see together the associations between Chakra, massage, and essential oil, in one of the usual practical summarizing charts:

Chakra	Areas to Massage	Essential Oils
1° Chakra	Buttocks, legs, and feet	Sandalwood, patchouli, and cypress
2° Chakra	Below the navel, the hips, and the base of the back	Jasmine, pine, and ylang-ylang
3° Chakra	Abdomen and stomach	Mint, black pepper, and cloves
4° Chakra	Chest and shoulders	Rose, sweet orange, and lemon balm
5° Chakra	The base of the neck and neck	Eucalyptus, chamomile, and verbena
6° Chakra	Face	Neroli, mint, and thyme
7° Chakra	Head and scalp	Olibanum, jasmine, and sandalwood

You will have noticed that some oils are effective for more than one Chakra according to the different characteristics that they possess. When you choose an oil to use always make sure to pick the scent you prefer, and with which you feel comfortable. This is the most effective way to obtain the best result. In fact, if you use an oil whose smell you don't truly like, you will end up with headaches and discomfort.

The connection between essential oils and Chakra, therefore, allows you to easily restore the balance of a Chakra at the moment in which this balance should fail. It also allows you to maintain a correct and constant flow of energy, take care of yourself, and maintain your physical, mental, spiritual, and emotional well-being.

You can apply this great method in total independence, fully enjoying its powerful results. There is one factor, however, that you must pay attention to when using essential oils to help your Chakras. It is the quality of the oils. Many oils on the market, especially the cheaper ones, are not pure and are not good for your Chakra healing journey. You must always make sure to buy pure oils. It is not difficult to find them, they are now widespread, and you can find them more or less everywhere. Before making your purchase be sure to carefully read the label where it is indicated the composition of the oil, to avoid wrong purchases. Also try to buy from stores that have testers, especially in the beginning. This will help you figure out if a fragrance is right for you and will prevent you from spending money unnecessarily. Since quality oils are a little more expensive than impure ones, it's best to buy something you're sure you'll use.

Before we move on to the benefits chapter, I'd like to close this section with one last piece of advice: only use one oil to start with. I know you may want to use this method right away to clear more than one Chakra and you are eager to try different oils but it is important to start slowly. You must try a single oil for a few days to understand how you and your body react to the fragrance and to this practice. If all goes well, you can begin to expand your selection of fragrances to use and continue to expand it over time.

The Power of Chakras: Benefits of Healthy Chakras on Physical, Mental, Emotional, and Spiritual Levels

Having open, healthy Chakras, free from blockages and with a balanced energy flow will allow you to enjoy a state of pleasant health on a mental, emotional, spiritual, and physical level. I think at this point in the book this concept is already clear to you. However, I would like to address in detail some of the greatest benefits that you will enjoy so that they can serve as a spur to begin immediately your path of analysis, healing, and maintenance of your Chakras.

Chakras' care is what we call holistic medicine. Holistic medicine takes care of the physical, mental, spiritual, and emotional aspects of a person at the same time; as opposed to traditional medicine which only treats one at a time according to the symptoms. If you suffer from any disease or have any health problems, you should always continue to take care of your body according to the medical prescription you get from your doctor. Studying and healing your Chakras can be a positive support to whatever path of healing and care you are following because it will take care of your emotions, your spiritual side, and your mental side, making the care of your body more efficient. This book is not intended in any way to replace medicine, but only to help you feel better, teaching you how to prevent discomfort, take care of your body, and always work in support of your well-being, through all the benefits that the energy of the Chakras can give you when it flows properly in your body.

Let's see together the main benefits.

You'll Feel More Positive

One of the first changes you will notice after working on your Chakras and balancing them is that you will feel more positive. When all the Chakras are open, healthy, and balanced, you are in a state of physical, mental, spiritual, and emotional well-being. This new feeling of overall wellness allows you to see everything in a new, more positive light. You will easily see the positive side of things. You'll understand people and their behavior better, so you won't distress yourself by seeing their actions as an attack on you. You'll be aware that sometimes things don't go the way you want them to but that soon the wheel will turn on your side. You will see this and much more. You will see your world and your reality with new eyes. You will finally see the beauty of the world around you.

You'll Be Less Sad

Having the Chakras in balance eliminates the sense of sadness and helps us to know how to deal with it when it arises due to a negative circumstance such as for example, the loss of a loved one.

When the Chakra energy flows correctly and without blockages, your vision of the world is so clear that you can understand that everything that happens to you happens for a specific reason. This awareness makes you live more positively, as I pointed out at the beginning of this chapter, and this removes the sense of sadness.

Moreover, when your Chakras are healthy and balanced, you are not blocked by stress or unmanageable, and out-of-control emotions, so you are not in danger of being overwhelmed by unmotivated sadness.

If at this moment, you are experiencing a sense of sadness because of a particular event in your life or for no reason, you need to work on the Fourth, Sixth and Seventh Chakras. The Sixth, and Seventh Chakras are particularly important in this circumstance because they influence your spiritual sphere and the relationship with a higher power that allows you to accept and deal with events that can bring sadness.

You'll Manage Anger Better

If each Chakra is well balanced, you will very rarely get angry, and if you do, it will be very easy to manage.

The regular practice of Chakra meditation and Yoga sessions will help you, more than any other exercise, to enjoy this benefit.

It is important to be free of the ballast of anger because it influences several negative factors in our lives. If you act out of anger and in anger, you will end up with personal, professional, and health problems.

The fundamental Chakra to focus on if you have problems controlling and eliminating anger from your life is the Fourth, the Heart Chakra. You will have to concentrate on your exercises to get its perfect balance. The Fourth Chakra influences emotions and its balance allows us not to be overwhelmed by them, or let them get out of control. In this way, you will be able to manage and eliminate anger.

You'll Sleep Better

The importance of sleep concerning a person's health has been underestimated for too long and it is only in recent years that studies on the subject are emphasizing its importance.

Lack of sleep or poor quality sleep negatively affects the state of our body, mind, and spirit. You've probably had a bad night's sleep and got up in the morning in a bad mood, with little mental clarity, a little sore, constantly hungry, and wanting to eat junk food. Think about what damage a stressful situation of the type just described can cause in your life, especially if it is repeated more or less frequently.

You'll be down in the dumps, in a bad mood, and maybe a little depressed. All the junk food will give you stomach problems and, probably, your skin will show unwelcome pimples. The lack of mental clarity will lead you, in the long run, to make poor choices and poorly reasoned, with all the precipitation of events that this can cause. From this situation of mental, physical, and emotional stress, your immune system comes out extremely tested, with all the consequences that this entails.

Fortunately, when Chakras' energy flows properly through your body and puts it in a state of total well-being, the quality and quantity of your sleep are no longer an issue. You'll sleep well for as long as your body needs. You will know this for sure, both because of the feeling of wellness you will experience, and because by following the exercises in this book you will have learned to communicate with your body, and listen to its messages.

The use of Chakras' meditation in any of its forms helps a lot to ensure the quality of your sleep. It puts you in such a state of well-being that your body will not find blocks or obstacles to falling asleep. In addition, meditation helps you to better dialogue with your body, and you will receive useful messages, in case you need to intervene in some way to further improve your sleep (That's why I have often repeated the importance of the last step of meditation, which is to analyze how you feel, before opening your eyes again).

Usually, it is the First, Third, and Fourth Chakras that influence sleep. If you find that the quality of your sleep is not adequate or you feel that you are not getting enough sleep, you could dedicate your Chakras' meditation in turn to these three specific Chakras, to rebalance their state of health. Alternatively, you can focus on one particular Chakra by identifying which one is causing the problem. The first Chakra affects sleep in general and its quality. If, however, you feel you don't want to sleep, the cause may be the Third Chakra. If instead, you feel very tired even at a mental level, but you can't sleep at all, the fault is of the Fourth Chakra.

Linked to this topic is the discussion about dreams. If your sleep problems are in some way related to dreams, then you must work on the Sixth Chakra, because the problem comes from the unconscious and it is the Sixth Chakra that deals with it. Take care of your Chakras to sleep well.

Only thanks to healthy and balanced Chakras will you sleep better and enjoy the benefits of better sleep, avoiding the discomfort, and stress that inadequate sleep causes in a person's life.

You'll Be Less Stressed

Doing exercises to maintain Chakra balance and practicing Chakra meditation regularly will help you gradually eliminate stress from your life.

Living a stress-free life brings a whole host of benefits, which you're probably familiar with, but are worth remembering.

First of all, as we mentioned earlier, being stress-free allows you to rest better, and see life in a more positive light. Stress often brings with it a sense of anxiety, a feeling of emotional blockage, and is also a real obstruction to achieving your goals, and what you want to achieve in life. Without it, you will be calmer, more emotionally balanced, and finally ready to get everything you want out of life.

So, practice daily all the methods you have learned in this book to keep your Chakras balanced and enjoy the benefits of a stress-free life.

You'll Manage Depression Better

When your Chakras are aligned and functioning well you will feel in control of your life and emotions, free from stress, energetic, bubbly, and full of zest for life.

When these elements are lacking in your life then you begin to feel a sense of depression. Depression comes from a feeling of lack of control over your life and your emotions. This sense of lack of control causes energy loss, apathy, weakness, and stress.

To manage the onset of a sense of depression you will need to focus your exercises on the First, Third, and Seventh Chakras. In a couple of weeks, you will begin to feel the first benefits. You will feel the energy that begins to increase, you will want to move and do physical activity. Stress will slowly recede from your life along with depression.

By keeping your Chakras in good health and perfect balance over time, you will be in continuous control of your life and these unpleasant feelings will become increasingly rare, even disappearing with the constancy in taking care of yourself.

You'll Have Healthier Relationships with People

When your Chakras are working at their best, you will feel at ease with people, stable balanced in their presence, and it will be easy to accept novelty and change in your relationships with them. You will be able to build healthy relationships with those around you without problems, you will know to whom to give your trust without fear, and you won't be overwhelmed by what you feel for those people.

Every relationship in a person's life touches so many points that all the Chakras end up being involved. Only the complete balance between all 7 Chakras allows us to live our relationships with others in the best way. A healthy relationship with others is fundamental to living our lives well. On the contrary, an unhealthy relationship brings with it negative energies along with all the consequences that negative energies cause in us, and in our lives.

By the term "relationship with others", I mean a relationship with a family member, a friend, or a partner. When we feel unstable with someone or we just can't trust even those who are reliable in a proven way, then we need to balance the First Chakra.

When the problems are in sexual or emotional relationships where we are too rigid and inflexible, then we need to balance the Second Chakra.

If emotions and confidence are unstable and, therefore, we become aggressive towards others then we need to balance the Third Chakra.

If we don't realize that we are loved and we can't feel the right emotions then we need to balance the Fourth Chakra.

If we fail to communicate with friends, family, or partners then we need to balance the Fifth Chakra.

If we cannot overcome differences of opinion, petty disputes, and disagreements with people around us then we need to balance the Sixth Chakra.

If we cannot think clearly and objectively and we act angrily when interacting with a person, perhaps excluding that person completely from our lives then we need to balance the Seventh Chakra.

As you can easily see by yourself, only a perfect balance of all 7 Chakras can allow you to have healthy and balanced relationships with people, and enjoy the benefits that this state brings. So, make sure to take care of your energy doors regularly to enjoy all the benefits that this balance can bring into your life.

You'll Be More Passionate

To fully enjoy life, it is important to live all its aspects with passion and appreciate all it has to offer.

By keeping your Chakras healthy and balanced with daily exercises and meditation, you will be able to live all aspects of your life with passion, such as your work, your family, your hobbies, and of course your relationship with your partner.

When your Chakras are well balanced you will see the world around you from a better perspective and it will be easier to enjoy what it has to offer. You will feel connected to this wonderful world, you will feel part of it, and ready for all the beautiful things it has in store for you. All of this will make you live your daily activities and your sex life with passion.

There is a close connection between the passion you put into your daily activities and the passion you experience in your bedroom. If you are going through a cold spell in sexual passion, take a look at your life, and, almost certainly, you will notice that you lack passion in a lot of other areas.

Get your Chakra energy flowing smoothly and balanced to enjoy the passion you deserve in all areas of your life.

You'll Achieve Your Goals

When your Chakras are healthy and their energy flows balanced, it is easier to get results, improve your performance, and achieve your goals. This happens because the state of well-being that we experience allows us to perform to the best of our abilities, without anything blocking, or hindering us. We feel so well that everything becomes easy to achieve.

There is no stress to hinder us, so we sleep well and feel good. This wellness allows us to have excellent performance in whatever area we are interested in, it allows us to build healthy, balanced, and positive relationships with the people we want in our lives. In addition, since we feel free from blocks, our self-confidence is very high, and this is an essential element to achieving personal success.

You'll Strengthen Your Body and Set in Motion a Prevention Mechanism

Our minds and our emotions act directly on our bodies. As I have repeatedly pointed out in this book, by taking care of your energy points, you will ensure mental, spiritual, and emotional health that will have beneficial consequences on your body and your physical health.

If you have never taken care of your Chakras until now, probably your emotional, mental, and spiritual conditions have somehow afflicted your body as well. You will see things change very fast when you become familiar with the DIY techniques to take care of yourself I shared with you in the previous chapter.

If, for example, you live in a constant situation of mental and emotional stress, you may be very overweight, always have a runny nose, a cold, a headache, or a constant sense of fatigue even when you do little or nothing. This happens because you sleep badly, eat poorly, waste energy because you can't think straight, and so on. I think you know very well what I'm talking about.

When your Chakras are open, healthy, functioning, and balanced, you experience such a positive emotional, spiritual, and mental condition that you lessen the negative repercussions on your body until they go away.

It has been scientifically proven that stress and depression damage your immune system, making you easy prey to bacteria and viruses that cause flues and colds, but also other diseases. The state of well-being you find yourself in when your Chakras are balanced, on the other hand, increases and strengthens the health of your immune system because you eliminate the damage caused by stress and depression in your life.

In short, by taking care of your Chakras with constancy you will set in motion a mechanism of prevention that will allow you to significantly raise the quality of your life. With your Chakras open and balanced you can take care of yourself by living a healthy life on a physical, mental, emotional, and spiritual level.

Conclusion

We have come to the end of our journey together and I would like to thank you for following me this far. Before letting you go, I would like to draw the conclusions from what we have said so far and leave you with some final advice and considerations.

In the first part of the book, you've learned the basics about the characteristics of each Chakra. At this point, you are perfectly able to analyze yourself physically, mentally, emotionally, and spiritually to understand where to begin your journey to open, unlock, and balance your Chakras. With the notions I have shared with you, you are able to associate your "symptoms" to the corresponding Chakra, and make your own "diagnosis". Now that you know which Chakra needs your attention, you can use all the DIY techniques shown in the second part of this book to open, heal, unblock, and balance it.

There isn't a Chakra more important than another one. To choose wisely the one to prioritize, you simply need to analyze your situation, how are you feeling now, and start from the areas that cause you more suffering and discomfort.

If you can not find a precise starting point, my advice is to start doing exercises for unlocking and rebalancing all the 7 Chakras, addressing them in order, from the lowest to the highest. The most efficient exercise that I recommend to you at this stage of confusion is "The 7 Chakras' meditation" which will allow you to see things in a clearer light. This technique will also give you the best results in the shortest time on all levels of your being: physical, mental, spiritual, and emotional.

Another piece of advice I would like to share with you is to create a Chakra routine for yourself. I used this method myself when I started to approach this discipline, and it helped me a lot. We, humans, are very habitual beings, and doing something new is always a bit complicated, especially at the beginning when we are not yet used to it. Building a routine and starting to practice it will help you to implement Chakra healing in your daily life.

Let me explain. Choose the practices that best suit you among those I have illustrated and begin to incorporate them into your daily routine, giving them specific spaces. My main problem was that I tended to forget new things, so I used sticky notes as reminders. Let me give you an example. I had arranged my house so that each different area was dedicated to a color, the prevalence of one color in a specific area of the house helped the corresponding Chakra. Also, I had taped on my closet and in the kitchen a chart where I assigned a color to each day of the week, and that day I dedicated clothing and food portions to that color. This was my method for using color therapy.

I had a list of 7 affirmations, one for each Chakra, that I kept taped to my bathroom mirror as a reminder to repeat them in the morning as soon as I woke up, and at night before I went to bed, so I wouldn't forget to use positive affirmations to balance my Chakras.

I had also created my own meditation corner at home, furnishing it with semiprecious stones and essence burners, as well as colorful rugs and fabrics. I had set reminders on my phone, at times when I was sure to be home, to remind me of meditation time, rather than massage, or stone therapy time.

It may seem a bit rigid and schematic at first, but it is the best method to develop the habit of taking care of your Chakras. In 3 or 4 weeks the habit will begin to consolidate and it will become spontaneous for you to perform various actions for your daily well-being. From that moment on, you will realize that the bar for the quality of your life will be raised a little higher every day, and you will probably no longer need sticky notes and reminders because taking care of yourself will become spontaneous.

Once you have unlocked your Chakras, don't let them get stuck again. Pay attention to your body's signals and the emotional, mental, and spiritual messages you receive in the form of intuitions. They will tell you immediately if a particular Chakra is about to get blocked, close, or get out of balance, and you can immediately intervene on it with one or more of the methods you have learned in this book.

My advice is to practice your Chakra routine daily, or at least as regularly as possible according to your schedule, to keep stable the balance you have obtained. This will prevent most of the future blocks and imbalances from occurring and keep you and your Chakras in a state of health and wellness.

Now we have truly come to the time of farewells.

I hope I have helped you in some way with my experience. I hope you have enjoyed this journey together and that it has been as enjoyable for you as it has been for me to accompany you in the discovery of the energy points of your body. Thanks for being with me and have a nice life

Namasté

Anja

Mind, Body, and Spirit Masterclass

www.ingramcontent.com/pod-product-compliance
Lightning Source LLC
Chambersburg PA
CBHW050248120526
44590CB00016B/2261